THE

Serotonin
Solution

TO NEVER "DIETING" AGAIN

THE
Serotonin
Solution

TO NEVER
"DIETING"
AGAIN

By

Robert B. Posner, M.D., Diplomate American Board of Internal Medicine, Founder and Medical Director of Serotonin-Plus Weight Loss Program

Contributors:

Donna L. Eckenrode, MPAS, PA-C, Serotonin-Plus USA Director of Clinical Training

Julia Yuskavage, M.S., R.D., Serotonin-Plus USA Director of Nutritional Programs

Lanalee Araba Sam, M.D., Diplomate American Board of Obstetrics and Gynecology, Medical Director of Elite Obstetrics and Gynecology in Ft. Lauderdale, FL

Joyce P. Hair, M.D., Diplomate American Board of Obstetrics and Gynecology, and Founder and Director of Cross Cultural Women's Health Issues, Inc.

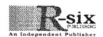

An Independent Publisher

R-six Publishing :::: worldwide

THE SEROTONIN SOLUTION

Copyright © 2014 Robert B. Posner, M.D.

Serotonin-Plus Weight Loss Program

Burke, Virginia

www.spdiet.com

Second edition

Cover design by Luanne Stevenson

Edited by William Zeisel

Printed in the United States of America

ISBN 978-1548435127

CONTENTS

1. Introduction

By Robert B. Posner, M.D.

This is an updated version of *"The Serotonin Solution to Never Dieting Again"*. The first version came out in 2010 and 7 years later, I would like to say that our first printing resulted in an earth-shattering, revelation-filled, awe-inspiring game changing intervention in the obesity epidemic. But alas, the nation's most serious health problem has only worsened. With all of the improved technology of smart phones, fit bits, health apps, improved diet drinks and a number of other positive developments in knowledge in science and nutrition, why are we losing the battle?

Stroll through the "health" section of a bookstore and you will be inundated with books professing to hold the "secrets" to easy weight loss. The books will display cutesy, fancy or funny titles, have lively cartoon pictures on the cover and feature quotations from Oprah or some other well-known celebrity telling you, "This is a great book to read."

I am sorry to inform you that this book holds no miraculous secrets. Its title isn't cute, it offers no cartoons of skinny women looking at food, and I have no clue whether any celebrity will read this book, let alone recommend it.

What I *can* tell you is that the information you will read in it is based on a reality approach to weight loss that has been carefully extracted from our vast experience at the Serotonin-Plus Weight Loss Program®. We have the experience of over

200,000 patient encounters both at our Flagship office in Northern Virginia and now in physicians' offices in 23 states of helping patients lose weight safely and effectively.

Our experience has taught us many things. One of them is that long-term weight loss requires a multi-dimensional approach. Any "fad" diet, "miracle" supplement or artificial meal-plan-based program is doomed to fail long-term. Many people can *diet* successfully, but they will succeed at long-term weight loss only if they change their lifestyles and behaviors.

Lots of work is required! That is a message you may not want to hear. But think of it this way: you are making the choice to invest time and effort in becoming healthier and thereby happier. It's a choice that will require the counting of portions from the different food groups, along with giving up some of the eating behaviors that you have grown comfortable with. It will also mean learning how to approach stressful situations in ways other than resorting to eating high-calorie foods. Overall, understanding that weight loss and maintenance require thought, focus and planning will go a long way in helping you achieve your weight loss goals.

Our nation must reverse the ominous epidemic of obesity. While the media focuses on swine flu, cancers and other scary illnesses, we are quietly experiencing one of the largest epidemics in our history. Not one disease state even comes close to approaching the magnitude of death and destroyed lives that weight problems cause Americans. It is estimated that by the year 2018, 43% of Americans will be obese, and we will be spending $343 *billion* dollars a year on obesity-related health problems.

What disease states are associated with being overweight? Let me count them or at least the most serious! I begin with diabetes mellitus, heart disease, stroke and blood clots. I continue with arthritis, cancer of the pancreas, stomach, colon, breast, uterus and esophagus, followed by sleep apnea, asthma, restless leg syndrome and dementia. And let's not forget the psychological issues: depression, poor self-esteem and self-confidence, despondency, withdrawal from friends and loved ones and avoidance of social situations.

A Book for Real People

This book was written to help people understand why it is so difficult to lose weight and then offer reality-based solutions. Our theories, case studies, solutions, recipes and tools have been developed from experience in treating thousands of people in the Washington, D.C., area. The people who have been through our program are not "clinical study" patients at some university or volunteers who are being paid by a pharmaceutical company. They are real people, just like you, who have tried virtually every fad diet that hits the news; who have lost hundreds of pounds over the years only to gain them back in yo-yo fashion; who consider having gastric bypass or other surgeries; who are facing significant medical problems because of their weight issues. And they are people whose self-esteem is in the gutter because of their weight problems.

Someone who has never experienced a weight problem may find it difficult to understand how people become overweight, and even more puzzling why they cannot lose the weight. Likewise, an overweight person might have difficulty understanding how the chronic gambler could lose house and family because of a destructive behavior pattern, or how the alcoholic could lose his/her livelihood because of chronic drinking. The following chapters will discuss some of the chemical factors that may be contributing to detrimental behavior patterns. However, chemicals (and their genetic basis) are just one aspect of this picture. Cultural, societal and familial factors also play a large role, and we will address them too.

Clearly, losing weight helps you feel better, live longer, rid yourself of medications, look better in your clothes and have more energy. This is truly a "no-brainer" situation. Your choice to lose weight is also a choice to be happier and healthier, but as you read through the following chapters, please keep in mind that success in achieving and maintaining your goal weight requires lifestyle changes. We all have spent years building certain behavior patterns, some of which may contribute to weight gain.

This book will provide an understanding of the causes of weight problems and will arm you with the tools to reach and maintain your goal weight. The following chapters describe the multifaceted issues involved with weight issues; they also include testimonials by people in our program who have been able to lose significant amounts of weight and maintain a lower goal weight. Through our experiences at the Serotonin-Plus Weight Loss Program®, we have identified a number of common behavior patterns and challenges and offer solutions that will be of great value to you in achieving your weight loss and maintenance goals.

2. Weight Control Basics

By Robert B. Posner, M.D.

Why Do We Want to Lose Weight?

Ask thousands of people why they want to lose weight, and you would get thousands of different reasons. Right? At the Serotonin-Plus Weight Loss Program we do just that. We ask every patient this question, "Why do you want to lose weight?" Surprisingly, we do not get thousands of different answers, only a handful. Our patients, who represent a wide range of demographics, give us four major reasons for wanting to lose weight.

1. *Health.* Most people understand that their weight issues are putting them at risk for serious medical maladies. Being overweight leads to an increased risk of diabetes mellitus, heart disease, stroke, peripheral vascular disease, degenerative arthritis, chronic back pain and breast cancer and other malignancies. Losing weight and maintaining that weight loss will markedly reduce their health risks.

2. *Vanity.* "Vanity" carries a bad connotation, but it really should not. There is nothing egocentric or narcissistic about wanting to look younger, have a higher level of confidence and self-esteem and receive favorable attention from those around us.

3. *Clothes.* Women will often complain about not fitting into the stylish clothes in their closets or wanting to buy clothes that are more form-fitting. Swimsuit season invokes much anxiety for fear of looking unsightly in summer wear. Losing weight helps us look and feel much better in clothes and allows us to select from a wider array of clothing styles.

4. *Energy.* Many of our patients describe a global sense of decreased energy and complain about being unable to keep up with their children. At home after a long day at work, they have little energy to exercise or do anything construed as fun, other than eating!

Interestingly, when men are asked why they want to lose weight, the health category is far and away the most common answer. Very few say much about vanity, clothes or energy.

In addition to these four main categories, our patients often mention two others.

5. *Occupational Needs.* Military personnel can have their career pathways put in jeopardy by being overweight. Promotions can be denied based on weights that are disproportionate to height. In the civilian sector, career advancement derailed by weight problems is not as openly detailed by policy, but numerous studies have shown a workplace bias against overweight individuals.

6. *Heightened Libido/Sensuality.* Most people feel sexier at a more optimal weight, and certainly impotence and other sexual dysfunction has been linked to obesity.

So the battle lines are drawn. The intellectual part of the brain tells us to lose weight for the aforementioned reasons. The instinctual part of our brain sets us up for the eating behavior patterns that are fun and easy, leading us to put on weight. What do most of us do when confronted by this collision of mind and instinct? We go on a "diet."

Basically, a diet means changing our eating behaviors for a period of time. As long as this change involves eating fewer calories or burning off more, we lose weight. As the weight starts coming off, we feel better, have more energy, look better in our clothes, and our friends and loved ones tell us how good we look. Bravo! We have crossed the finish line. The diet is over.

We then start (slowly at first) migrating to old behavior patterns. Why? Because they feel good. However, the weight starts coming back, and we are back on the yo-yo. The result? Incredible frustration!

How can we stop this seemingly never-ending sequence of events? Why are some people able to lose weight and keep it off while others seem to be destined for the yo-yo?

Why Is It So Difficult?

You go to your physician's office for a refill of blood pressure and cholesterol medications, and the nurse weighs you. The doctor walks in, looks at the chart and says, "You need to lose weight."

Well, tell me something I don't know! (WTMSIDK!)

If your physician takes this discussion one step further, you may hear, "Eat less and exercise more."

WTMSIDK!

And, if the physician wants to offer more advice, you will hear, "Eat more protein and fewer carbs."

WTMSIDK!

Here is something you *do* know: It is very hard to lose weight despite mentally understanding what you need to do to achieve the weight loss. Obviously, taking in fewer calories than you burn will result in weight loss. There are two ends of this equation: your dietary intake and your exertion activities. To lose weight, you need to intervene, preferably on both ends of this equation, meaning, eat less and exercise more. If we know this is what it takes, then why is it so difficult to follow through?

This is what I tell my patients. We humans are naturally "wired" to be a weight-gaining species, not a weight-losing organism. It is more "natural" to eat and gain weight than monitor our food intake and lose weight. What do I mean by this?

Let's first discuss the taste of food. What tastes best to our palates, high- or low-calorie foods? If I blindfolded 1000 adults and put a carrot stick in each one's mouth and then a piece of cheesecake, 999 would tell me that the cheesecake tastes much better. Do you ever crave a great piece of lettuce, or does a glass of water calm you down after a long day at work? If you are like 99% of people, you crave chocolate and yearn for that glass of wine at the end of your day.

Another issue that compels us to eat as opposed to limiting our calories involves the use of food as a reward system. As a child, if you behaved, you got ice cream. If you finished your plate of food, you were allowed to have dessert. Likewise, as adults, we tend to reward ourselves with high-calorie foods. At the end of a long day or week, we feel that we deserve something good. Among the quickest and most inexpensive rewards are a good glass of wine, a fine restaurant or a tasty dessert. Sure, there are other ways of rewarding ourselves, such as a day at the spa, a new outfit or tickets to a great show or sporting event, but they are not immediate gratifications.

The slowing of our metabolic rates with aging is another reason why it is so difficult to lose weight. It affects females much more than males, especially for women who have gone through childbirth. How many of you remember being in high school or college and eating three times the amount of food you eat now, consuming much more alcohol, but weighing much less than you do now? Years ago, you didn't need to count calories or worry about desserts, and you probably didn't even have an exercise program. Now, putting on weight is almost indecently easy.

And then there are the holidays and special occasions. When we get together with family and friends, no matter what the culture or nationality, a big meal is the centerpiece of the event. For my family's celebrations, we gathered at the dinner table, not at Gold's Gym. My grandmother was insulted if I didn't eat at least three plates of food at our holiday events. Christmas and New Year's, a vacation week, a birthday party or other celebratory event — an overabundance of food is the rule.

Humans tend to gravitate to things that feel good and move away from things that don't. What feels better: sitting with friends, having some drinks and dinner and discussing life's events, or going to a gym with those same friends and running on a treadmill? I don't think I have to answer that question.

Here is another example of how human nature can sabotage weight loss efforts. You go to a very expensive buffet brunch that offers more types of food than you can count, including a famous dessert bar. Who makes one trip to the food bar and doesn't return? Everyone goes back for seconds, thirds or more. You paid for this, so get your money's worth!

I often give my patients this role-play. I am a famous Hollywood producer and you are a famous movie star. I am paying you $10 million to play the lead role in my picture and I call you into my office and say, "I need you to *gain* 10 pounds by the end of the month to better portray the character in the movie." What is your immediate response? Easy or hard to do? Next question: Will you have fun doing it? The answers are obvious. Now let's switch the situation. I am the producer and I am asking you to *lose* 10 pounds in the next month. What are your initial thoughts? Difficult or easy? Fun or not fun doing this? Again, the answers are obvious.

"It's Not My Fault"

You have seen the television commercials for weight loss supplements, telling you that your weight problem is not your fault. It is stress that's making you release hormones that cause you to retain fat.

You are at your family reunion and you notice that almost every one of your cousins, aunts, uncles and other relatives is overweight. You conclude that your weight problem has been dealt to you by the genetic cards.

You are entering a certain time of your monthly cycle, in which you have uncontrollable cravings for something sweet. The M&Ms are calling you by your first name. Despite trying hard not to be consumed by thoughts of these sweet little candies, you are driven to plow through an entire bag.

At times, it seems that the destiny of our own weight is somehow interfered with by cosmic forces beyond our control. We all know that to lose weight we must eat less and exercise more, but we feel stymied in our efforts. Let's address these issues individually.

The release of stress hormones like cortisol, epinephrine and norepinephrine takes place under "fight or flight" situations. If you have ever been in a near-accident situation and felt your heart pumping, you understand this reaction. However, no rigorous studies demonstrate that fat deposition, obesity or the inability to lose weight are related to the normal fluctuations of these hormones.

Familial factors like a history of weight problems can be a predictor of future weight issues. Our individual metabolic rate, number of fat cells and satiety mechanisms will differ according to genetic predisposition, but the family environment may play a more significant role. Every family unit has its own traditions relating to eating behavior. For example, do your first memories of family gatherings also call up images of sugar-laden "treats" being placed in front of you? Were you made to feel guilty if you didn't have at least three oversized portions of Granny's homemade meals? If your good behaviors were constantly being rewarded with high-calorie foods, that pattern will likely extend into your adult years.

Regarding the irresistible cravings for chocolate and other sweets during certain times of the female cycle, the cause lies in brain chemical imbalances, most notably of serotonin. I will provide a fuller discussion of brain chemicals and how they affect weight, mood and other behaviors in the following chapter.

Taking ownership of your weight situation is a very important step in attaining your goals. Even if you were dealt genetic and environmental cards that are not optimal, you can still play a winning hand. There is no "fault" here: not your family lineage, not your internal chemicals and not some self-perceived personality issue.

Instead, think in terms of a multi-factor scenario that consists of genetics, environment, and, for whatever reason, a natural predisposition for human beings to be a weight-gaining species. If human beings were meant to be ideal weight organisms, wouldn't a carrot stick taste better than a piece of cheesecake? Wouldn't it be really fun to snack on water and cucumbers instead of a piña colada and a creamy dessert? Gaining weight is easy and enjoyable, and losing it is difficult. This is no one's fault, it is reality. The sooner we face this reality and stop blaming, the sooner we can get down to the work necessary to win the battle.

If It Sounds too Good to Be True...

To quote P.T. Barnum, "There is a sucker born every minute." Infomercials! Among the most entertaining times for watching TV are the early morning hours. In case you have not experienced insomnia, you are missing an incredible array of entertaining shows that make weight loss seem so easy. Tune in and you will find:

Talk-show formats where an "expert" praises a pill that magically allows you to shed many pounds while eating the foods you like. You will even see people crying into the camera as they tell you how this little pill changed their life forever and ever.

A *New York Times* best-selling author (and former prison inmate) ranting psychotically about how "they" do not want the general public to know about natural cures, pills and other methods of natural weight loss.

Ex-professional ballplayers and actresses telling you how they lost over 50 pounds eating the incredibly delicious prepackaged foods offered for sale.

All of these programs have something in common. If you buy their products, books or foods in the next 10 minutes, you get an unbelievable deal–free meals, free diet books, free newsletters and perhaps even a free bottle of the magic pill!

The direct response industry is clearly one of the biggest scam businesses in America. The marketing agencies putting together these campaigns know that those of us who want to lose weight crave a simple, easy answer that allows us to eat the foods we want. The infomercials and commercials offer a shortcut that does not require diet and exercise.

The Federal Trade Commission has been clamping down recently on products that claim to cause significant weight loss without dietary intervention and exercise. Why? Because they do not work alone. *There is no such thing as a pill that makes you lose weight without appropriate diet and exercise.* If there were, a major pharmaceutical company would have patented it and been offering it by prescription. Do not be fooled by claims that a pill can block cortisol and offer easy relief from belly fat.

Recently, the television personality, Dr. Mehmet Oz was hauled in front of a Senate committee to explain why he promoted many products, such as Green Coffee Beans, to the public, claiming that these pills produced easy weight loss. Dr. Oz was chastised by the committee members for using his TV show (and forum) as a vehicle to promote products that dupe the public.

Also do not be fooled by claims that a conspiracy by the pharmaceutical companies or the United States government is concealing "natural weight loss cures." If you Google the authors of books that detail these conspiracy theories you will find an interesting array of infomercial hucksters, whose resumes include FTC fines, prison time and absolutely no credibility in the weight loss arena.

The commercial programs that sell you prepackaged foods try to hook you by showing pictures of actresses and sports heroes "before" and "after," and telling you how much weight they lost. I am a guy from the 70s and I loved it when Tony Orlando sang "Tie a Yellow Ribbon," but I would bet that when he finished his contract with the sponsoring company, he went back to his old eating patterns and regained lots of that 100-pound weight loss.

Eating prepackaged foods is only a temporary change in behavior patterns, and as soon as you go back to "real" food, you will most likely go back to old patterns. At our clinics, we encourage patients to eat real food because that is what they will be eating for the rest of their lives. For long-term success in weight control, you need to learn how to eat the correct proportions of the different food groups. Opening up a package of food does not teach that behavioral change.

The bottom line is this: there are no shortcuts to long-term weight loss. Even the bariatric surgeries are not a panacea, as we have had many patients come into our program months after their procedures because they start gaining substantial weight again.

I offer this image to my patients. The reasons why we want to lose weight are the pot at the end of the rainbow. The trip along the rainbow is a difficult one, lined with saboteurs trying to knock us off course. The well-intentioned family member giving us chocolate for the holidays, the jovial friend reassuring us that those few drinks can't possibly hurt our weight loss efforts, our own internal chemicals imploring us to eat food when we feel stress...all of these are barriers in our quest to lose that dreaded extra weight and keep it off.

Remember that another saboteur is the huckster promising "easy, effortless" weight loss. There is a sucker born every minute. Do not be one!

"I'm a Stress Eater"

When people think of stress, the immediate reaction is usually a negative one. The picture emerges of a sweaty, anxious, heart-pounding, gut-wrenching reaction to some really bad work or personal issue. Stress is something we loathe, something we try to avoid, something we inherently know will hurt us both physically and mentally. We fear stress and will try hard to avoid stressful situations.

Sometimes, however, stress can be a good thing, propelling us to the very limits of our performance capabilities. An example of this would be a professional athlete competing in a high-stakes game before thousands of people in the stadium and millions more on television. Watching athletes like Michael Jordan, Tom Brady or, ahem, Bob Posner compete on the intense national stage (okay, for Posner it's Springfield, Virginia) shows that stress can heighten performance.

Stress-Induced Binge Eating. At the Serotonin-Plus Weight Loss Program, a common theme among our patients is "stress" or "emotional" eating, which is characterized by reaching for food that provides immediate gratification. The binge foods tend to be high-calorie snacks such as candy or chocolate, and we reach for them in small, repetitive "treats" like chips, nuts or M&Ms.

Stress-induced binge eating is followed by self-loathing for having given in to a deleterious behavioral pattern. We know that eating these food sources only temporarily mitigates some of our stress and anxiety. Conversely, the weight gain from stress-induced eating behavior actually worsens stress and makes us feel more anxiety. We enter a vicious cycle that hinders us from losing weight.

Why do many people turn to high-calorie foods as a "treatment" for stress and anxiety? Is this a learned response or some type of chemical-based, reflex-type of action? What can we do to recognize and avoid this behavior pattern?

To some extent, we have been taught to medicate ourselves with food when we are not feeling well. Think back to your childhood. When you were upset about something, your parents would calm you with some ice cream or other treat. We often equate nurturing with being provided with food.

From a chemical standpoint, eating carbohydrates will provide a temporary boost in the production of *serotonin*, sometimes called the "feel good" body chemical. When serotonin levels are depleted, such as during times of significant stress and anxiety, the brain sends out chemical signals causing us to seek out the foods that contain the building block for serotonin. This building block is an amino acid called *tryptophan*. Unfortunately, the food sources that contain tryptophan are chocolates, carbohydrates and other high-calorie food sources. In the next chapter, I will discuss serotonin and other body chemicals affecting our weight.

Resisting the Eating Reflex. Recognizing the chemical and environmental contributions to stress-induced binge eating does not, by itself, stop that behavior. We feel compelled toward this behavior pattern, as if some force of nature controls us. How can we avoid giving in to the almost reflex-like detrimental eating response?

It would be easy for me to advise patients to convert "negative" stress to positive stress by exercising, lifting weights or working out with a punching bag. Physical activities dissipate muscle tension, burn off calories and elevate our stress-fortifying "fight or flight" hormones. However, eating that Twinkie sure seems like an easier, quicker and less sweaty response to stress.

Look at it this way. The body has many reflexes, and basically, a reflex is a reaction that takes place without the person thinking about it. When a physician hits your knee with a reflex hammer, your leg will jerk involuntarily. However, if you concentrate on your leg and tense up, the reflex reaction may be substantially less intense. When people are confronted with stress or other negative events, many will turn to eating, almost as a reflex. To break this reflexive behavior, you have to find some way of delaying the reaction.

One suggestion is to ensure that damaging food sources are not readily available where the stressful situation is taking place. Suppose you are working under deadline on an important project, and your boss is breathing down your neck. You feel your heart pounding, you are stressed to the max, and in your desk draw is a bag of M&Ms, your favorite snack (especially the blue ones). You intend to eat only a few, but when you close down for the night, that bag of M&Ms is empty. Oops!

The obvious solution is to *not* have the M&Ms in your desk. The less readily available the detrimental food source, the less likely that you will eat it. Similarly, in the house, ensure that the food sources that you tend to binge on, like chips, nuts, ice cream or chocolates, are not in the cabinets. When you go shopping, buy only the foods on a list you generate before going to the store. (And do not put M&Ms or Twinkies on that list!)

Another tactic is forcing a time delay between the stressful situation and the eating behavior. At Serotonin-Plus Weight Loss, I often advise my patients to keep a 3x5 card with them that contains, in bullet points, the five major reasons they want to lose weight. Whenever they feel compelled to eat high-calorie food as a response to stress, they take out that card to review their reasons. If they still feel they need to eat the food, they must first turn the card over and date and initial it. By taking several minutes to delay and think about the reflexive eating behavior, they may avoid the dietary indiscretion.

Diverting yourself with more healthy activities is certainly another way of addressing stress and anxiety. Taking a brisk walk while listening to music, playing a competitive game such as racquetball or tennis, working in the garden and other diversionary activities will allow you to avoid the caloric intake from stress-induced eating and also to burn off calories. The contracting and relaxing of muscle groups is actually a very good way of dissipating stress. Yoga, meditation and Pilates are also activities that help address stress in a healthier, adaptive way.

The reflex-like reach for food and/or alcohol is difficult to break. However, we can learn to regain control of our emotional-eating behaviors and reach our goal, if we learn how to control the stress, not let the stress control us!

Conclusion

The bottom line is that human beings are configured more to be weight-gaining than weight-losing creatures. That is why it is so difficult for us to lose excessive weight and even more difficult to keep it off. Achieving and maintaining an optimal weight is possible, but only if we understand the key factors and are not sucked in by programs, books, supplements and fads that purport to make weight loss simple and easy.

3. The Serotonin Connection

By Robert B. Posner, M.D.

Why Serotonin?

We named our program *Serotonin-Plus Weight Control* because so much of what governs our moods, eating behaviors and feelings of satiety is a result of chemical balances and imbalances. Among all the chemicals in our body, serotonin is one of the most important for any discussion of weight gain and loss. Serotonin was discovered during the 1930s in the lining of the gastrointestinal tract, in blood platelets and also in the brain.

After it was recognized, in the 1950s, that serotonin functions as a neurotransmitter (chemical messenger for the nerves), a tremendous amount of research was performed to understand the role of serotonin and its receptors in various physical and psychological diseases. The total body content of serotonin is between 10 and 12 milligrams, about 1/30th of the weight of one regular aspirin tablet. Amazingly, such a small amount has profound effects on appetite, mood, memory, learning, sleep, cardiovascular function and a number of other essential body functions.

Serotonin imbalance has also been linked to depression, anxiety, bipolar disorder, panic attacks, migraine headaches, premenstrual syndrome (PMS), postpartum depression, seasonal affective disorder, irritable bowel syndrome and carbohydrate cravings.

How Serotonin Works

How can one chemical, present in minute amounts in the brain, have so many different clinical implications? The answer involves the different receptors that exist for serotonin in the brain, cranial arteries and intestines. If you want to dive into the details of serotonin and its receptors, I recommend a book, *Doctor, I Have a Chemical Imbalance: The Serotonin Story* (written by a shameless self-promoter named Robert B. Posner, M.D.).

The production of serotonin requires the availability of tryptophan, an amino acid found in many natural food sources, including turkey and chicken, and also in carbohydrates and sweets. Tryptophan is first converted to 5-HTP, a serotonin precursor that has been used for mood enhancement and appetite suppression. Once 5-HTP is formed, another series of reactions converts it to 5-hydroxytryptamine, or 5-HT, which is serotonin. Certain nerve cells are involved with the storage and release of serotonin.

Many prescription medications work indirectly via serotonin mechanisms. Anti-depressants such as Prozac, Zoloft and Lexapro raise serotonin levels at one type of site (1-A receptors) involved with mood modulation. These medications contain no serotonin. Instead, they elevate serotonin levels by inhibiting something called the "transport carrier." They carry the tag "SSRIs" standing for Selective Serotonin Reuptake Inhibitors. Several other antidepressants such as Effexor, Cymbalta and Pristiq work via serotonin mechanisms and other neurotransmitter regulation. There are serotonin receptors in the cranial (head) arteries, and several migraine headache treatment medications work by stimulating those receptors. Imitrex, Relpax, Zomig and Amerge are medications in this class.

The brain and the intestine contain another type of serotonin receptor that is involved with cravings for carbohydrates and the sensation of feeling full. Animal studies show that rats fed serotonin orally seem to have an earlier level of satiety and decreased food intake. This finding helped prompt my research on oral serotonin supplementation in humans and the development of the serotonin formula that is used in our weight loss centers.

The explanation for carbohydrate cravings is not completely known, but here is a likely scenario. When serotonin levels are depleted, the brain sends out signals that make us seek foods that contain tryptophan, the building-block of serotonin. Since tryptophan is found in high levels in carbohydrates, we feel compelled to eat high-carbohydrate foods. Females tend to have more carbohydrate cravings than men, since they are more prone to serotonin deficiency; they are also more prone to develop diseases associated with serotonin deficiency, including migraine headaches, irritable bowel syndrome and depression.

There are a number of other brain and body chemicals involved with satiation and cravings. Leptins, ghrelins, cholecystokinins, glucagon-like peptides and insulin are just some of these natural body chemicals involved in eating and satiation. Pharmaceutical companies have been attempting to develop drugs that intervene with these chemicals in ways to help either reduce appetite or enhance satiation. Success has been very limited.

Development of Serotonin Supplementation

As a physician practicing internal medicine, I have seen numerous patients with serotonin-imbalance conditions, most notably depression. I have prescribed serotonin-altering medications, but the success rate according to the literature and my clinical experience is no more than 66%. This response rate is only 10% above placebo! My mother, now deceased, suffered from severe depression that failed to respond to virtually every prescription antidepressant on the market. To see the suffering that occurred in my mother, and also in my father who lived with her through years of mental disease, helped prompt me to search for a better type of intervention.

I began my search by asking: If serotonin precursors like 5-HTP are being used to promote increased production of serotonin, why not provide the active ingredient itself? Why can't we just give oral serotonin supplements? My literature search gave me an immediate reason for pause.

Like a medieval castle, the brain is surrounded by a protective moat, called the blood-brain barrier, and the medical literature I was reading said that serotonin in the bloodstream cannot pass across it. However, as I reached deeper into the literature, I found no definitive proof that serotonin cannot cross the blood-brain barrier. I did find studies demonstrating that when oral serotonin was fed to rats, their eating behaviors changed. Other studies showed that when serotonin was injected intravenously into cats, their behaviors changed. How could these changes be explained if the blood-brain barrier prevented serotonin from reaching the receptors involved with these behaviors?

I concluded that serotonin probably does penetrate the blood-brain barrier, and that if I could protect the oral serotonin molecule from degradation in the bloodstream, I might be able to get enough of it into the brain. But before the serotonin supplement got into the bloodstream it would have to pass through the stomach, which is simply a churning pouch of acid. I feared that digestion would degrade the serotonin and make it useless. (That is why, when you pile tryptophan-rich foods like bananas and walnuts on your hot fudge sundae, you can't claim you are trying to raise your serotonin levels!)

One way to avoid the breakdown of a chemical in the acidic environment of the stomach is by using an enteric-coated capsule. However, I needed to know how much of the serotonin would remain intact after passing through the stomach. Since I could not find any literature about the stability of serotonin in an acidic environment, I performed a study. My colleagues and I put the serotonin molecule into an environment simulating gastric acid and then measured to see how much remained. After three hours in this acidic environment, the serotonin was mostly still intact. We then heated the serotonin and the simulated gastric acid to 150 degrees F for up to 45 minutes. The serotonin remained stable. We had discovered that serotonin is not destroyed by stomach acid.

After the serotonin passed through the stomach it would enter the intestine and then the bloodstream. Our next puzzle was to control events in the blood. Serotonin is metabolized in the bloodstream by the oxidizing enzymes monoamine oxidase (MAO) and aldehyde dehydrogenase, which render the serotonin molecule ineffective. My colleagues and I used antioxidants to prevent this metabolic breakdown.

Testing for Safety and Effectiveness

Once the formulation was developed, we performed an animal safety study to ensure that the direct use of oral serotonin supplementation would not be harmful. During these safety studies, we made a fascinating discovery. The serotonin concentration in the brain of beagle dogs was measured around 0.4 nanograms per deciliter. Keep in mind that a nanogram is 10 to the minus ninth of a gram, which is an incredibly small amount. This vitally important brain chemical is present in minute amounts, comparable to scooping up a handful of sand on Waikiki Beach. What effect would our supplement have on this exquisite chemical balance? Our safety studies demonstrated that even at 100 times the human serotonin dosage, eight-pound beagle dogs exhibited no significant adverse reactions to the serotonin product.

I was awarded a U.S. patent (Number 6,017,946) for the serotonin invention in January 2000. This allowed for continuing development of a product and commercialization of the concept.

The next step was to perform human studies with the Serotonin-Plus® supplement. Unlike a major pharmaceutical company that has millions of dollars for research, we performed an independent study through a weight loss physician in the Springfield, Virginia, area who was paid per patient regardless of the results. A double-blind, crossover, placebo response study was performed on 35 people. Study participants had to take Serotonin-Plus for 6 weeks, then placebo for 6 weeks, making the study a "crossover" model. The use of a crossover model allows each person to act as their own control, meaning that variables, such as age, environmental factors, and other concomitant medical issues do not need to be considered, making the findings of the study more reliable. Additionally, neither the patients nor the physician knew which 6 weeks they were on the active product versus placebo, thus making the study "double-blinded." The patients were seen every 2 weeks for a weigh-in and blood pressure check, and completed a questionnaire about other symptoms such as mood changes and energy issues. They also met with a physician, but were not given any specific program to follow, just general dietary information.

The study results demonstrated that during the active Serotonin-Plus treatment phase, there was a 0.8 pound weight loss difference per week when compared to placebo. While a weight loss of 0.8 pounds per week may not seem aggressive, it was statistically significant in comparison to placebo. If you extrapolate the average weight loss per week out over the course of 6 weeks, or in the case of our current program of 12 weeks, this equates to an additional weight loss over placebo of 4.8 pounds and 9.6 pounds for the 6- and 12-week programs, respectively. In other words, the serotonin supplement accounts for almost 10 pounds of weight loss over the course of a 12-week program.

Moreover, there were statistically significant changes seen in the mood and energy parameters, showing that during the Serotonin-Plus treatment phase, mood improved and energy levels rose. There were no significant side effects.

Establishing the Program

When my studies demonstrated safety and efficacy, I decided to write a protocol for a weight loss program with the serotonin supplement, also incorporating a prescription anorectic medication, a dietary plan and weekly visits. I wrote the protocol because, as a practicing physician, I knew that lifestyle changes are the key element to losing weight and maintaining that weight loss, and taking a pill does not constitute a lifestyle change.

The program began at my medical practice in October 2002, and since then over 23,000 patients have gone through the program at all of our centers nationally. The average weight loss in the 12-week protocol is 30 pounds for females and 40 pounds for males, and some patients lose much more. We have generated excellent diabetes prevention data as well as helping many people reduce or actually obviate their needs for diabetic medications.

How much of the success is due to the serotonin supplement as opposed to the prescription medication, office visits and other support? Determining that is not particularly significant because we are not offering our product as a "take this and lose weight" supplement. When you look at the studies on the prescription medication alone, the average weight loss is about 1.2 pounds per week. The Serotonin-Plus program averages 2.5 pounds of weight loss per week. Is this because of the accountability of the visits? Is it due to the serotonin supplement? The bottom line is that the serotonin supplement is a component of a comprehensive program that is helping many people lose weight safely and effectively.

Serotonin supplementation has other benefits too. Many patients tell us that they experience positive effects from the supplement, including mood enhancement, increased energy, heightened libido, decreased frequency of migraine headaches, fewer PMS symptoms and diminished anxiety.

Concerning depression, the prescription antidepressants work via one or more of the three major neurotransmitters implicated in mood disorders: serotonin, norepinephrine and dopamine. Some antidepressants, such as Prozac, Paxil, Zoloft and Lexapro, work to raise serotonin at one type of receptor site by inhibiting a transport carrier involved in the removal of serotonin. We have had many patients successfully transition from their prescription serotonin-affecting medications to the natural serotonin supplement. However, it is important for an individual to check with their own physician before discontinuing a prescription medication.

Some migraine headache sufferers report a diminished frequency and severity after the use of the supplement. Migraine headaches are due to the dilation of blood vessels in the brain. Serotonin receptors on the walls of the cranial arteries are involved with the regulation of the diameter of these vessels. Certain precipitating factors such as the menstrual cycle, changes in the weather, ingestion of foods with monosodium glutamate (MSG) and stress can cause dilation of the cranial vessels, resulting in a migraine. A group of prescription medications called triptans attach to the serotonin 1-D receptors and activate them just as serotonin does. The resulting vasoconstriction of the arteries reverses the process that causes the migraine headache. Federal Trade Commission laws prohibit dietary supplements from claiming the prevention or treatment of disease, so we cannot state definitively in this book or on the bottle that the serotonin supplement prevents migraine headaches.

Many patients who have experienced PMS symptoms, seasonal affective disorder and menopausal-associated depression, all caused at least partly by serotonin imbalance, report that their symptoms improved with the natural serotonin supplement. Once again, we have not performed any controlled studies about this, so the reported benefits are "anecdotal" as opposed to being demonstrated in a pharmaceutical-like double-blind, placebo-controlled study.

Conclusion

Serotonin is present in minute amounts in the body but has a powerful impact on many key bodily functions. We at Serotonin-Plus Weight Control have discovered how to use a natural serotonin supplement as a part of our highly effective and safe weight loss program.

4. Who is to Blame for America's Most Significant Health Issue?

By Robert B. Posner, M.D.

A Growing Crisis

Under the watch of our federal, state and local health departments and healthcare officials, America's obesity epidemic has been spreading almost like a cancer. The ramifications include spiraling expenditures on hospitalizations, medications and surgical procedures, lost time at work and early death. In some regions, such as Indian reservations, the diabetes incidence exceeds 50%, and the obesity problem contributes greatly to this.

The facts are ominous:

- In the United States, it is estimated that 93 million Americans are affected by obesity.

- Individuals affected by obesity are at a higher risk for impaired mobility and experience a negative social stigma commonly associated with obesity.

- Socioeconomic status plays a significant role in obesity. Low-income minority populations tend to experience obesity at higher rate and are more likely to be overweight.

- Almost 112,000 annual deaths are attributable to obesity.
- In the United States, 40 percent of adults do not partici-pate in any leisure-time physical activity.

Below is a map of the obesity rates by state in 2013. If this were compared to the same map from 1985, you would be shocked to see just how much prevalent obesity is now compared to almost 30 years ago.

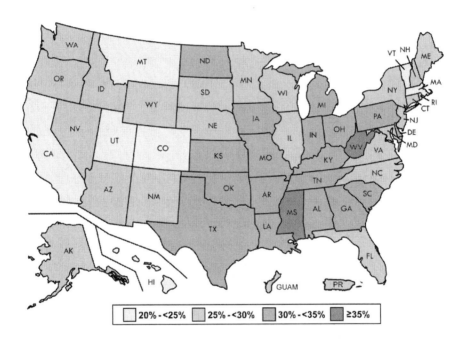

If we think our healthcare expenditures are completely out of control now, as the baby boomers (born between 1948 and 1964) age, healthcare costs will far exceed our ability to pay for them. Does this mean some type of rationing of care? Do we deny dialysis to people over 80? Do we not treat certain cancer patients aggressively?

The Causes of the Obesity Epidemic

The alarming increase in obesity can be traced to a number of contributing factors. The recognition of these forces will lead to a better understanding of how we can approach the problem from a number of different angles.

Society and Culture. Showing people how much we love them by feeding them an extraordinary amount of food crosses all religions, races and cultures. Almost every event is based on eating food, and lots of it. Think of your holiday dining room table covered by more food than could possibly be consumed by your family and guests. We are almost made to feel that we are insulting our hosts by not filling up our plates.

But take a moment to think this through with me. If one of your friends or relatives was a known alcoholic, would you give him/her a bottle of vodka as a show of love and caring? If one of your friends was a known drug abuser, would you give him/her a needle and a fix for the holidays as a way of showing your affection? Of course not.

Now answer this question. If being overweight leads to an increased risk of heart disease, cancer and premature death, why would any loved one hasten the development of these life-altering events by forcing food on us? Whether a frost-laden chocolate cake for our birthday, freshly baked cookies for Christmas or Grandma's special pudding, our loved ones always seem to reward us with high-calorie foods. For the overweight person trying to lose weight, this sabotages efforts to achieve a healthier status.

Clearly, as a society intent on helping each other live longer, healthier lives, we all need to be cognizant of how we recognize our family and friends during holidays and celebrations. We all need to learn how to show love and caring in ways other than providing calories to someone who will be hurt by their weight situation.

Corporate America. Does the CEO of a huge company selling you prepackaged foods really care whether you maintain your weight loss? Does that famous has-been star hawking those same products think about what's in your best interest? Do our friends at the chain burger joints think lots about the cholesterol plaque building up in your arteries, caused partly by the poor diet of most Americans?

The answer to these questions is a resounding No! Large public companies and their CEOs have to answer to their shareholders and board members. Often, profit is the major motivation and successful performance is gauged more in terms of how much profit is made as opposed to how many people have truly been helped. These CEOs would not want to intentionally harm people, but the advertising and marketing of huge burgers, beer and sugared sodas are contributing to the growing problem of obesity. There is nothing illegal about the marketing, sales and advertising of high fat/high calorie foods. The consumer has a choice of eating healthy or supersizing their fries, but the slick commercials, the special deals and targeting our children with toys and cross marketing with their favorite movie are all ways of influencing our eating behaviors. The advent of cable and satellite television has resulted in hundreds of channels being available at our fingertips, and the plethora of commercials extolling the virtues of double stuffed cookies and mouth-watering burgers and fries is extremely influential on eating behaviors.

The Training of Primary Care Physicians. Medical schools and residency programs often lack emphasis and focus on preventive medical care. Nutrition, psychology and human behavior courses are not given the same importance as other disciplines, and therefore, young physicians enter the medical field more adept at treating illnesses than preventing them. The curriculum committees at medical schools and post-graduate training programs must start implementing a much more aggressive approach about weight problems that will prepare physicians to intervene effectively. Courses in nutrition and the psychosocial aspects of eating behaviors should be required in the early years of training, and continued during the residency.

Insurance Companies. Everyone has a story about the predatory nature of health insurance companies, from the denial of necessary services to not paying claims on time to forcing changes in prescribed medications based on the approved formulary. As a physician, I have found health insurance companies to be driven by profits and the bottom line. It is easy for them to deny or stall your claims, engage "review" physicians who will not approve your MRI or other diagnostic test and keep lowering the fees they will pay your physician for services at the same time they are increasing your premiums.

Preventative care? To go back to my New York City roots, *Fuggetaboutit!* Insurance companies will pay for prescription medications for hypertension, diabetes, or high cholesterol, but refuse to reimburse for treatment of obesity, which is often the cause of these maladies. The costs of hospitalizations and interventional procedures would greatly diminish if patients achieved weight loss prior to the onset of the later stage medical *sequelae.* You would think insurance companies would recognize this and jump on the weight loss bandwagon, but in reality they provide little, if any, support to people who need and want to lose weight. One of the reasons why is that historically, people only remain with a particular insurance company for only several years. The "investment" by an insurance company in the *future* health of a person will not save that insurance company money in the future, because the chances are that the person will no longer be covered by that company. The savings will be realized by some future insurance company covering the patient, and that company was not the one that made the preventative "investment".

The insurance companies make another, less obvious contribution to our obesity crisis when they reduce reimbursement rates that physicians are receiving from managed care. Doctors must see more patients to generate the same revenues, thereby cutting into the time they can spend with each patient. Very few primary care physicians can afford to talk about behavior modification. Moreover, the decreasing insurance reimbursements do not allow for the physicians to hire nurses and/or assistants to provide counseling and intervention for effective weight loss.

The Government. The federal and state governments are spending money on healthcare initiatives, but there has not been a coordinated effort to reverse the trend of rising obesity rates. Displaying pamphlets about good nutrition on the racks of local libraries is nice, but ineffective. Starting at the schools, there must be more aggressive education and commitment to teaching our youth about the dangers of obesity.

The Recession. During difficult economic times, many families have less money for food. Recent data suggest that almost one-quarter of the children in the United States are not receiving as much food as they should because of tight family finances (a mind-boggling number). This is the United States, after all, not some third world country.

When monetary resources dwindle, parents are apt to feed their families with the lowest cost food items available. You can buy more calories per dollar at a fast-food burger place than at a "healthier" restaurant. Concerning the preparation of "home-cooked" meals, high-calorie food sources such as pasta and high-fat meats are a bargain compared to foods that might be less likely to cause weight gain. Additionally, restaurant choices may be altered because of a tighter budget. Therefore, one result of the recession has been an increase in the prevalence of obesity.

Conclusion

At our weight loss centers, we strive to help our patients with individual accountability as well as factors that may be beyond their control. By identifying these contributing external influences and our internal control systems, we are more likely to reverse the ominous trend of an ever-increasing weight problem in America.

5. African-Americans and Weight Loss

By Lanalee Araba Sam, M.D., and Robert B. Posner, M.D.

Scope of the Problem

As an African-American obstetrician/gynecologist who has battled with weight and body image issues since childhood, I, Lanalee Araba Sam, feel uniquely qualified to assist Dr. Posner with this essay and with his clinical mission to combat obesity. Dr. Posner deserves credit for soliciting my contribution and acknowledging that as a slim, fit, Caucasian male he may not be the ideal authority on this subject. On the other hand, my personal experience as a previously obese African-American female provides me with a deep understanding of the factors that challenge African-American women and our overweight community in general. Now that I have introduced myself, I will join Dr. Posner in laying out the facts and discussing the issues associated with obesity and the African-American community.

The following data clearly reveals the severity of today's crisis. Consider the following unfortunate statistics:

- African-American men are 30% more likely to suffer from heart-disease-related death than non-Hispanic whites.

- African-Americans are twice as likely to be diagnosed with type 2 diabetes as non-Hispanic whites.

- African-Americans are 1.7 times as likely to have a stroke as non-Hispanic whites.

The data for African-American women is just as troubling:

- Roughly 4 out of 5 African American women are clinically overweight or obese.

- Based on having a body-mass index (BMI) of 30 or more, 61% of African American women aged 60 and older and 53% of those aged 40-59 are classified as obese.

- From 2003 to 2006, African-American women were found 70% more likely to be obese than non-Hispanic white women.

The statistics are shocking, but the magnitude of this problem becomes even more disturbing when other significant weight-related causes of death are also considered, such as breast, colon, stomach, pancreatic and esophageal cancers.

Causes

Clearly we need to understand why obesity is affecting the African-American community so much more than non-Hispanic whites, and what can be done to reverse this life-threatening situation. Several objective factors are believed to contribute to the disturbing statistics cited above. Weight problems in any group of people are influenced by a number of interrelated factors: genes and biochemistry, home and environment, socioeconomic status, cultural norms and corporate behavior — which I will now survey.

Genes and Biochemistry. Whether it is the color of our hair or eyes, our risk of developing cancer or the speed of our metabolism, genes play a large role in who we are and what we look like. The African-American patients that I see complain that everyone in their family is overweight. Does this mean that they are doomed by their genetic heritage to be overweight in spite of efforts to control their body weight? I will address this issue in more detail a little later.

Numerous chemical mediators affect eating behavior patterns. A serotonin imbalance, for instance, may lead to cravings for carbohydrates. Alternatively an imbalance of leptins, another class of chemical messengers produced in the body, may affect how and when we feel full after eating. The science remains imperfect, but it is safe to say that other chemical imbalances are also involved in the eating/hunger/satiety process and may contribute to an increased risk of obesity. Chemical imbalances that predispose to obesity may be more prevalent in the African-American community, but because these chemicals are present in minute amounts, there is no simple way of measuring them through blood testing or MRI/CT imaging. Consequently there is no definitive way of testing the chemical imbalance hypothesis as the explanation for obesity. Fortunately, we can overcome the potential impact of these factors with education, nutrition, exercise and health-conscious diligence.

Home and Environment. The contribution of home and environment to weight issues cannot be overemphasized. African-Americans typically grow up in households where almost all family functions are centered on the consumption of delicious but very high-calorie foods. At family events, not to consume excessive amounts of food is tantamount to insulting the cooks, who take understandable pride in the feasts they prepare.

Most of our African-American patients tell me that when they were growing up, there was very little emphasis on healthy eating habits and weight-conscious nutrition in their households. The most commonly consumed foods were rich in calories, and portion control was never emphasized. Many of the traditional Southern dishes in particular are notoriously high in fats and carbohydrates. Needless to say, constant exposure to such an indulgent food culture is not conducive to being at a healthy weight, and because eating patterns are typically endemic to the family, most if not all of the members of a family become overweight.

Socioeconomic Status. Numerous studies have shown that although it has been steadily improving, a significant disparity still exists between the African-American community at large and white Americans in terms of advanced schooling and income levels. African-Americans achieve less affluence than their white counterparts, and those in lower socioeconomic groups tend to place less emphasis on education and nutrition. The combination of having fewer resources available to purchase healthier food choices, plus less understanding about how and why it is important to do so, means that many African-American households are stocked with higher-calorie, less nutritious daily fare. Outside of the home, too, there is insufficient attention paid to proper diet. School curriculums seem woefully deficient in mandatory courses that teach children proper nutritional guidelines and how to embrace a healthy lifestyle. This contributes directly to the childhood and adult obesity epidemic.

Cultural Norms. As much as we may not like to admit it, because we don't want to be considered shallow, most of us care about what others think of our external appearance and are influenced by societal standards of attractiveness. This social pressure is considerably greater on women than men, since you cannot ignore the ubiquitous media images of slender models and actresses presented as the ideal of feminine beauty. Supermodels strive to be a size zero and will take every step necessary to not put on any weight. Consequently most "regular" women feel that in order to be seen as attractive they must also conform to these thin standards. However, many African-American men find a curvaceous body type more attractive than the waif-like Caucasian ideal. Rap music artist Sir Mix-A-Lot's entertaining anthem "Baby's Got Back" clearly declares this preference. The argument could be made, therefore, that because African-American women are appreciated for their ample curves, they are less concerned about monitoring their diets and their physiques. While they may not consciously desire to be overweight, the greater social acceptance that they enjoy from African-American men as attractive larger women could lend itself to bodies that devolve from sensually Rubenesque to sadly obese.

Corporate Behavior. Corporate America with its eye on the bottom line has successfully (and understandably) used the science of marketing to target susceptible groups of people with advertisements to convert them into paying customers. Certain high-profile hamburger restaurant chains, for instance, run catchy commercials directed toward prospective African-American consumers. With the increase in national obesity rates running parallel with the growth of fast-food franchises, it is clear that advertising is contributing to a major health problem. In the movie *Supersize Me*, which chronicles the experiment of a man who eats only "supersized" meals at McDonalds for an entire month, after one month this unconventional scientist and "food martyr" sees his weight balloon, his cholesterol level rise dramatically and his liver show signs of dysfunction.

Of course, no one eats every meal at Mickey D's, but the point is that frequent consumption of most fast-food items will result in significant weight problems and the concurrent development of other potentially life-threatening health conditions. There is nothing illegal about advertising, and the corporate forces behind them would probably argue that their restaurants now offer patrons a variety of "healthy" menu items such as salads and fruit. In reality, however, too many people carrying too much excess bodyweight purchase too much unhealthy food from these inexpensive dining institutions. Moreover, if communities with large African-American populations are infested with easily available fast-food options and few healthier alternatives, resisting the sweet and salty charms of these franchises in the name of weight control becomes even more difficult.

Solutions

As physicians, community leaders, educators, parents and politicians, we must all make a more focused effort in combating the obesity epidemic in the African-American community. Here are our thoughts.

Genes, Biochemistry, Home and Environment. African-Americans need a better understanding of weight-related issues, and that requires a sustained educational effort. Health and dietary education needs to start at home with young children and continue in the schools. Parents are wholly responsible for providing their children with proper nutrition, and if their children learn to be happy with unhealthy food choices early in their lives, this pattern will most likely continue into adulthood. The first step in breaking the pattern is to educate parents and caregivers about the serious medical complications associated with obesity. Providing free community health screenings and educational seminars at the workplace, churches and community centers can disseminate important nutritional information to adults that may result in healthier food and lifestyle choices for both themselves and their dependents.

The next step is for the schools to teach children the importance of maintaining a healthy body weight. Nutritional education of some sort needs to be incorporated as a meaningful part of the standard curriculum from elementary upwards. We fully appreciate the importance of algebra, language arts and other core academic subjects, but learning how to eat and exercise to maintain a healthy body weight and ward off disease is at least as important as learning how to solve complex mathematical problems or recite the periodic table.

Perhaps the most important result of greater education would be to provide an understanding that our genetic makeup does not make being obese inevitable. The characteristics we inherit may predispose us toward something, like sneezing during the pollen season or putting on weight, but we have methods to counteract these tendencies. Just as we can take medication to relieve sneezing, we can act to keep our weight under control or, if it is already excessive, bring it down to a healthier level and keep it there. That is an important message that must be brought to forefront of the African-American community's attention.

Socioeconomic Status. Although we cannot wave a magic wand that would put African-Americans at the same income level as

Caucasians, we can address a serious socioeconomic factor that greatly affects health and longevity. Studies show that African-Americans receive less health care than most others. We hope that the recent government overhaul of U.S. healthcare includes substantial funds and a meaningful policy to address the obesity epidemic, especially in the populations most affected. Government-funded weight loss centers could be established and promoted in African-American communities, for example, in conjunction with increased health education initiatives. This could help to address the disparity in access to and use of healthcare, especially as related to obesity issues.

Cultural Norms. The cultural acceptance of excessive weight, especially for women, needs to be challenged by those of us who are public and cultural leaders. Popular African-American politicians, clergy and other influential leaders have historically been very passionate and vocal in addressing important issues that affect our community. However, it is only with the election of President Obama that a major leader has paid meaningful attention to the most important single health crisis affecting the African-American population today, obesity. It is past time for community leaders to become more active and aggressive in promoting viable measures of intervention.

Corporate Behavior. It may be unrealistic to expect the fast-food empires to alter a profitable pattern of enterprise, but it would be a welcome change to see advertising that promotes healthier food choices, especially to customer groups like African-Americans. Alternatively or additionally, these companies could invest more in developing appealing menu items with reduced saturated fat and carbohydrate content.

Conclusion

The African-American community is experiencing a serious health risk for the development of debilitating and life-threatening medical problems at rates much higher than the Caucasian population. The incidence of type 2 diabetes is especially alarming, and if left unchecked will contribute to an exponential rise in associated illnesses such as stroke, heart attack, vascular disease and arthritis.

6. Weight Loss and the Menopausal Female

By Robert B. Posner, M.D., with Joyce P. Hair, M.D.

A Frustrating Situation

Clearly, not everyone with a weight problem in America is a female in the menopausal age range. However, we wanted to devote a chapter to this group because at our clinics we have found incredible frustration in perimenopausal and menopausal women who want to lose weight. Countless women over age 40 have said, "No matter what I do, I cannot seem to lose weight." Why is it seemingly impossible for them? Is it caused by estrogen deficiency? Does serotonin play a role? What strategies can help a woman over 40 attain her weight loss goals?

A woman's transition to menopause includes a period of time referred to as the perimenopause, a term in common use only since 1995. Perimenopause is the time when the ovaries begin to make lower levels of hormones, including estrogen, progesterone and testosterone, resulting in irregular periods and other menopausal symptoms. Actual *menopause* may start five to eight years after the onset of perimenopausal symptoms, and is defined by the cessation of menstruation for one year.

During the early stages of menopause, the ovaries start secreting less and less estrogens. The pituitary gland in the brain recognizes this and starts releasing more Follicle Stimulating

Hormone (FSH) and more Luteinizing Hormone (LH) in the attempt to stimulate the ovaries to produce more estrogen. On laboratory blood testing, the early stages of menopause will show a slightly low serum estrogen level and slightly high FSH and LH levels, and then as menopause occurs, these lab values become more elevated.

A woman can develop a number of life-altering symptoms during perimenopause and menopause. The more subtle ones include sleep disruptions, night sweats and decreased cognitive abilities like short-term memory lapses, faulty word recall, and decreased ability to concentrate; only to be followed by hot flashes, decreased libido, vaginal dryness, hair loss, weight gain and symptoms of depression and anxiety. As many of these symptoms mimic a low thyroid (hypothyroidism) condition, patients often present to our internal medicine practice with some or all of these symptoms, convinced that they have a thyroid problem. Laboratory testing usually demonstrates normal thyroid levels.

Depressive symptoms range across a spectrum, from mild to intense. They may include lack of energy, sleep problems, eating disorders, unexplained musculoskeletal pains, difficulty getting out of bed in the morning and lack of interest in hobbies or activities that used to be engaging or bring joy. More severe symptoms are feelings of low self-esteem, withdrawal from friends and loved ones, pessimism about the future and crying spells

Chemically, the question arises as to why the declining levels of estrogen lead to these depressive symptoms. The answer is the association of declining estrogen levels with a reduction in brain serotonin levels. Studies have shown that the brain uses estrogen to produce serotonin. Serotonin is made from a protein called tryptophan, and estrogen promotes the availability of tryptophan in the brain. During times of estrogen deficiency, such as the week prior to menses in the younger woman, when she may experience symptoms of premenstrual syndrome (PMS), or during perimenopause or menopause, the reduction of serotonin levels leads to depressive symptoms.

Treating the menopausal woman with hormone replacement therapy (HRT) does help the vaginal dryness, hot flashes and most other symptoms of menopause, but the mood changes may not be adequately treated with hormones alone. Many women are placed on prescription anti-depressants because their symptoms of depression are life-altering. Selective serotonin reuptake inhibitors, such as Lexapro, Zoloft and Prozac, are usually a first-line approach. (See Chapter 3 for a more detailed discussion.)

Factors in Combination

The perimenopausal or menopausal woman's difficulty in losing weight is most likely due to a combination of factors. A woman's metabolism slows down dramatically at this time in her life. Not only is it difficult for her to lose weight, but it is much easier for her to gain weight. Studies indicate that women using estrogen-based hormone therapy gain less weight and less fat than those who do not. Furthermore, short-term hormone suppression has been found to cause a decrease in resting metabolic rate of 40 to 70 calories per day, which would result in weight gain if not accompanied by a compensatory decrease in food intake or increase in physical activity. Even though she may consume fewer calories than she did in her 20s and 30s, the menopausal woman often still puts on weight due to slowing of her metabolism.

In addition to the changes in metabolism, the menopausal woman also experiences mood swings that affect her eating habits. Many perimenopausal or menopausal women change their eating patterns because of depression or anxiety. Some will turn to alcohol as a temporary escape from sadness, melancholy or sleep disorders. Unfortunately, alcohol brings weight gain, which further exacerbates the depressive symptoms. A truly vicious cycle begins.

Often, an individual will eat in response to stress, anxiety or depression. The woman experiencing menopausal depression may find herself reaching for chocolate, candies, excessive carbohydrates and other high-calorie food sources. This will also result in unwanted weight gain and the onset of a negative cycle.

Women transitioning through menopause may also confront situations that challenge a healthy dietary pattern. During their younger years, many women are so busy with work and raising their families that they have little time for social gatherings that provide alcohol and high-calorie foods. Later, once the kids are driving themselves around, attending college or otherwise do not need custodial attention, women may have more free time to attend after-work functions, "Sex in the City" parties and other social functions that may derail weight-control efforts.

Conclusion

The combination of chemical and hormonal changes, a slowing metabolism and social changes during the menopausal years can result in weight gain that seems impossible to control. We have found at our clinics that a diet high in protein and vegetables and low in carbohydrates and fruits, supplemented with serotonin, has a very positive effect on weight loss. The Transitional Diet Plan™ of the Serotonin-Plus Weight Loss Program will be discussed in Chapter 9. Its recommendations will guide you to success in reaching your weight loss goals.

7. New Weight Loss "Pills"

By Robert B. Posner, M.D

There is much excitement when the media pounces on the opportunity to report about a new "weight loss pill" that receives FDA approval. Why the excitement? Because almost 100% of the 68% of Americans with weight control problems would love nothing better than a "pill" that will solve the weight issues. Who wants to count calories, cut back on carbohydrates, reduce alcohol consumption and (heaven forbid) wake up one hour earlier to get exercise in before the work day begins? The specter of just swallowing a pill and seeing the weight shed off quickly and easily...well, that is worthy of all of the media coverage and excitement.

I am sorry to be the bearer of bad news, but here goes: there is NO "pill", whether the pill in question is an FDA-approved "weight loss" drug or an over-the-counter dietary supplement that will produce long standing weight control. Medications and supplements need to be viewed as adjuncts to what is truly required: Lifestyle/behavioral modification changes as this relates to dietary food and beverage consumption as well as exercise.

After seeing thousands of patients, I have observed that the "speed" of weight loss is important initially. When people embark on a weight loss/weight control journey, there is nothing more discouraging than getting on that scale and seeing ¼ pound loss that week, ½ pound or even 1 pound in a week. After trying week after week and seeing the results be 2, 3 or 4 pounds in one month? Discouraging to the point of getting into the "I give up" mindset. However, if the person sees 10, 15 or more pounds of loss in one month, there is an amazing positive energy that sets in because all of a sudden the "look" is much younger/healthier, the person has much more energy, clothes that have been sitting in the closet for years now fit, there may be medications that are not needed anymore, other people start complimenting the person, etc.

I believe that the prescription medications for weight control have a place in helping the patient get started and seeing fairly immediate results. If a doctor prescribes one of these medications and does not offer a structured program, including a "real food" dietary plan, exercise guidance and periodic support/accountability visits, there is little-no chance of that patient losing weight and keeping the weight off. If behavioral modification is not achieved, after the medication is finished, all of the weight will return. This scenario plays out over and over again, i.e. yo-yo dieting, when medications are used without structured support.

The prescription FDA-approved "weight loss" medications fall into different categories. Some work by suppressing appetite, others by blocking fat absorption and some medications work via other hormonal pathways that regulate food intake. Here are the common FDA-approved "weight loss" medications prescribed by physicians:

Phentermine

This medication has been FDA-approved since 1959 but it got its best notoriety when it was combined with another "weight loss" medication, fenfluramine. This combination was termed "Phen-Fen" and major problems became recognized in the mid-1990s. A number of women taking this combination of medications developed valvular heart disease and others developed a lung/heart problem called primary pulmonary hypertension. This resulted in the need for intensive medical treatment and in many cases, surgery to correct the heart valve problems. When the FDA and medical community investigated this thoroughly, it seems that Fenfluramine ("Pondimin" and "Redux" were the tradenames) was the culprit causing the heart valve issues. This drug was taken off the market and lawyers had a field day suing the manufacturers to the tune of $6 BILLION dollars worth of settlements. (Yes, that was Billions, not millions.)

When the dust settled, phentermine, which was FDA-approved in 1959, remained on the market and is probably the widely prescribed appetite suppressant. Phentermine is in the class of drugs called "amphetamines" and its' mechanism of action is by increasing metabolism and decreasing appetite. It is commonly prescribed at 15 mg-37.5 mg a day. Studies show an average of 1.7 pounds per week of weight loss when using this medication. Side effects of phentermine include sleep difficulty, dry mouth, constipation, elevated heart rate and agitation. The Serotonin-Plus Program utilizes phentermine in our protocol. I choose phentermine as opposed to any of the other FDA-approved medications due to the almost 60 year history of usage, and my literature review prior to devising the SP protocol clearly pointed toward phentermine as being the safest and most efficacious drug to use.

My "take": When used selectively in medically screened patients AND used as part of a structured weight control program, phentermine can be a very useful adjunct in allowing people to see a rapid enough weight loss response to keep them engaged long enough to allow the behavioral modification techniques to take effect.

Qsymia

This medication was approved for use by the FDA in July, 2012. Qsymia is not a "new" drug at all, but rather, a combination of two old FDA-approved medications: phentermine and topiramate (also known as "Topamax"). We already discussed the phentermine component so let's turn our attention to topiramate. Nicknamed "Dopamax" by physicians because of the disorientation sensation that a number of patients exhibit during the use of this medication, topiramate was originally released as an anti-seizure medication. The drug has also been useful for migraine headache prevention. However, at higher dosages, many patients noticed weight loss that occurred. When looked at specifically for weight control it is still not exactly clear how topiramate works to help lose weight but here are some potential mechanisms of action:

- Works on "addiction centers" of the brain to reduce the pleasure of food
- Reduces appetite
- Produces disorientation causing a person to forget to eat (You gotta love this dysfunctional mechanism of action)
- Alters certain hormones, including *leptins,* a hormone noted to affect appetite
- Loss of taste sensation

The average weight loss for people taking Qysmia is close to 10% of body weight after one year of treatment. The higher dosage form (15 mg of phentermine/92 mg of topiramate) results in more weight loss than the lower dosage (7.5 mg phen/46 mg topiramate).

The side effects of Qsymia usage include:

- Fatigue

- poor sleep
- disorientation
- bowel changes
- dizziness
- numbness
- memory difficulties
- altered taste sensations.

My "take": LOTS of side effects that may be experienced by the user and, if not used in combination with a structured weight control program involving behavioral modification, the use of this drug is ultimately not worth the time, money spent seeing doctors and the sacrifice of putting up with the adverse reactions that are experienced.

Belviq (Lorcaserin)

This drug was approved by the FDA for patients' usage in June, 2012. The mechanism of action involves the stimulation of certain types of serotonin receptors in the brain (sorry for the boring biochemistry, but here goes: the 5-HT 2C receptors) that are involved with appetite regulation. The average weight loss seen in patients using Belviq is about 4% of body weight. The usual dosage of 10 mg twice a day has not been shown to produce any of the heart valve issues seen with other prescription medications that worked via artificial serotonin pathways (the "bad" Fen).

Side effects of Belviq include:

- mental problems,
- slow heartbeat,
- headache,
- dizziness,
- drowsiness,

- feeling tired,
- fatigue,
- nausea,
- dry mouth,
- cough,
- back pain,
- constipation,
- painful erections,
- diarrhea,
- vomiting,
- upper respiratory tract infection,
- runny or stuffy nose,
- urinary tract infection,
- muscle pain,
- sore throat, or
- rash.

My "take": When reviewing the side effect profile, seeing the potential of a 4% body weight change and realizing that without a structured program being delivered along with the medication there is pretty much a zero chance of long term weight control, this would not be a recommended treatment option.

Contrave (Combination of bupropion and naltrexone)

Contrave was approved for usage by the FDA in September, 2014. Similar to Qsymia, Contrave is not a "new" drug, but rather, a combination of two older medications that have different indications. One of the components, bupropion (brand names "Wellbutrin" and "Zyban") works by affecting two brain chemicals: dopamine and norepinephrine. The original indication for bupropion was for depression (Wellbutrin) but then studies also showed a positive effect on smoking cessation (Zyban). The other component of Contrave, naltrexone, has been shown to reverse the effects of opioids and has been used to help people withdraw from opioid and alcohol dependence.

Concerning naltrexone, this is an opiate receptor antagonist and was originally approved by the FDA to help people with heroin addiction. This expanded into other opiate addictions as well as alcohol dependence. Specifically focusing on "weight loss", naltrexone has several possible mechanisms of action: Reduction of appetite, increasing metabolism, allowing the brain centers to delay immediate gratification behaviors and possibly, the weight loss comes from people drinking less alcohol.

The other component of Contrave, bupropion, has been shown in studies independent of the combination with naltrexone to help people lose weight. The mechanism of action is not exactly clear but may involved dopamine receptors and a lessening of cravings. Additionally, the improvement of mood noted with bupropion may result in more energy and time devoted to exercise.

The results seen with Contrave are modest at best. Studies demonstrate about a 5.4% body weight loss and this compares to about 1% for placebo. The potential side effects include: nausea and vomiting, constipation, headache, dizziness, insomnia, dry mouth, diarrhea, elevated blood pressure and heart rate and seizures. Moreover, because bupropion has been linked to the onset of suicidal thoughts, Contrave carries the same "black box" warning about suicide as seen on products containing bupropion.

My "take": When warnings occur about an increased risk of suicide and we are looking at a 5% body weight loss with little-no chance of long term weight control if behavioral changes are not permanent, it seems to make very little sense to use Contrave in a long term weight control effort.

Saxenda (Liraglutide)

Saxenda received approval from the FDA for use in 2014. This drug was released initially under the name *Victoza* as a treatment for diabetes mellitus. Saxenda is in a class of medications called "GLP-1 peptides". Basically, this drug mimics a natural intestinal hormone called "glucagon like peptide". One of the roles of GLP-1 is to tell the brain that you are full. Additionally, GLP-1 has affects on insulin that in turn, can result in weight changes. Saxenda is administered by a daily self-injection.

Saxenda provides between 5-10% of body weight loss. The list of side effects is extensive and include: low blood sugar;, nausea (especially when you start using liraglutide), vomiting, stomach pain; upset stomach, loss of appetite; headache, dizziness, tiredness; diarrhea, and constipation. There is a laundry list of previous medical conditions that preclude the use of Saxenda and patients are warned to immediately to their physicians if any symptoms develop while using this drug. The cost of using Saxenda approaches $1000 a month and most insurance companies are not covering its' usage.

My "take": One grand a month, 5-10% of (most likely non-sustained) body weight loss, numerous potential side effects and the need for self injections all add up to a pretty obvious recommendation: Spend the money on a personal trainer, home gym equipment, natural/healthy foods or a mortgage for a condo in Florida.

Xenical/Alli (Orlistat)

I am not going to spend much time discussing Xenical, which has been FDA for over 20 years. First released as an FDA-approved prescription medication, Orlistat became an over the counter consumer product in 2007. The mechanism of action involves blocking fat absorption. The reason why I will not devote much time to writing about Orlistat: The obesity rate has increased dramatically since the introduction of this fat blocker and the people that have benefitted from its' usage are ones owning interests in laundry/cleaning companies due to the soiled underwear that is prevalent in users of the product.

8. Serotonin-Plus Patient Pearls of Wisdom

By Robert B. Posner, M.D.

Learning from Our Patients

We have helped thousands of patients lose weight successfully and safely. Not only do patients learn lifestyle modifications from us, but we also learn a lot from our patients. We have learned that everyone is different. Sure, there are similarities in behaviors associated with weight gain or failure to achieve weight loss, such as stress-induced binge eating, mindless eating of repetitive foods and eating on the run (just to name a few). But there are many different approaches with subtle nuances that individuals take in order to change these detrimental eating patterns.

We asked our patients to give us helpful comments and tips, some fairly obvious and others more creative, as to what makes for successful weight loss. Hopefully, you too can learn from them. I want to thank our Serotonin-Plus Weight Loss patients for writing this chapter for us!

Our String of Pearls

1.   A sedentary lifestyle is part of my weight problem, so I added a frameless elliptical under my desk so I can pedal throughout the workday. No excuses about not being able to go to the gym! – *Mary M.*

2. Add cinnamon to your low-fat plain yogurt. It not only adds a great flavor, but cinnamon is a natural appetite suppressant as well! — *Anonymous*

3. Always eat the protein and veggies first in a meal and only eat a carb if you are still hungry. — *Anonymous*

4. Always go shopping with a list of foods to purchase and do not buy any item that is not on your list. — *Anonymous*

5. Always keep a pair of tennis shoes and socks in your vehicle, in case you find you have some extra time and want to take a walk or run! — *Anonymous*

6. Ask yourself before eating a detrimental food source whether you really feel "hungry." — *Anonymous*

7. Avoid alcohol. Not only does it provide empty calories, but it stops your metabolism in its tracks. — *Anonymous*

8. Avoid the chips and bread baskets at restaurants. — *Marcella S.*

9. Avoid thick dressings and sauces. — *Anonymous*

10. Blue plates are the least appetizing. I always serve my dinner on a blue plate. — *Anonymous*

11. Bring a cooler with diet-friendly food when you have a road trip. That way you avoid fast-food temptations. — *Anonymous*

12. Buy an outfit you really like that you can't fit into and look at it daily. It's a great motivator. — *Anonymous*

13. Buy vegetables in small packages; that way you don't have to eat the same vegetable every day for a week. — *Janet S.*

14. Buy your phentermine at Costco, it's cheaper. – *Connie B.*

15. Carrots are great to eat with salsa instead of chips. – *Celeste W.*

16. Chew sugar-free gum when you get a craving! – *Anonymous*

17. Clean out all the bad foods from your kitchen, so you're not tempted to eat the wrong foods. – *Connie B.*

18. Combine protein with fiber to fill up. Example: carrot sticks with low-fat cheese. – *Anonymous*

19. Cut your cheese in silly shapes, it makes it more fun to eat! – *Anonymous*

20. Do not eat after 8 p.m. – *Anonymous*

21. Do not eat small, highly repetitive, high-caloric food sources such as nuts, chips, popcorn, etc. – *Anonymous*

22. Do not eat when you are distracted: if you are at your desk working, watching a sports event at home or otherwise involved in some other activity. Distracted eating leads to over-eating and eating the wrong types of foods. – *Anonymous*

23. Do not go to "all-inclusive" vacation resorts where there is no limit to the amount of alcohol and food you may consume. – *Anonymous*

24. Do not go to "all you can eat" buffets. – *Anonymous*

25. Do resistance exercises while you watch TV in the evenings, like crunches, push-ups, lunges, and squats. – *Anonymous*

26. Don't be afraid to inquire about the menu at an upcoming event (e.g. holidays, parties or business affairs), so you can plan ahead. *– Anonymous*

27. Don't buy things that say "weight control" or "sugar-free" at the grocery store; they cost more and usually aren't better for you. *– Anonymous*

28. Drink 6-8 glasses of water a day. I start with my first cup shortly after rising in the morning and drink another every two to three hours during the day. Usually I have a half-liter (size of a small Perrier bottle) at each meal, which honestly is not very difficult to drink! People drink super-sized sodas with more ounces! And, those caffeinated drinks (which are diuretics) will make trips to the restroom frequent as well and are not healthy for you! *– Ina R.*

29. Eat every three hours (healthy snacks) rather than the common diet mentality of starving yourself. *– Lisa K.*

30. Eat fresh berries/fruit instead of dried, to cut down on sugar intake. *– Anonymous*

31. Eat sliced pickles; they are crunchy and salty like potato chips, but Phase One friendly. *– Anonymous*

32. Eat slowly and chew your food completely before swallowing. *– Anonymous*

33. Eat vegetable cheese; it has more protein and less fat. Plus, kids like it too. *– Annelle F.*

34. Exercise consistently. Power walk! *– Monica M.*

35. Exercise outside as much as possible. Try doing cardio using multiple routes with different elevations; it makes things much more interesting. – *Anonymous*

36. Find a friend or friends who are also trying to lose weight, and establish some type of friendly competition to crown the "Biggest Loser." – *Anonymous*

37. Find a partner to work with you on weight loss at the same time…spouse, friend or co-worker. It is easier to adhere to a dietary/exercise regimen when you have company. – *Anonymous*

38. Find day-to-day motivation. When you see results from setting and achieving smaller goals, it's easier to stay motivated. – *Pam M.*

39. Find the things you truly like to eat that are within the diet so you are more willing to stick to the plan. – *Lily P.*

40. Freeze a sliced banana for a small sweet treat. – *Anonymous*

41. Get a craving? Brush and floss your teeth. – *Carole H.*

42. Go to every follow up visit! – *Anonymous*

43. Hang out more with friends who do not eat or drink excessively. – *Anonymous*

44. Have a (low-calorie, low-carb) protein bar handy and don't forget to exercise! – *Nancy Jo N.*

45. Hungry late in the evening? Hot cup of decaf green tea sipped slowly…. is warm and comforting. – *Carole H.*

46. I keep a garbage bag in my closet so if I get bored and want to eat, I go try on clothes. Anything too big gets

put in the bag for charity. The added boost and visual reminder of how well I'm doing is better than a cookie any day! – *Mary M.*

47. I reclaimed control of my life and weight because I adopted the Serotonin-Plus "no negativity" attitude, which really helps! – *Antonia C.*

48. If I have a bad craving I promise myself that if I still want that particular food the next day I can have it, and then I forget about whatever bad food it was that I wanted. – *Anonymous*

49. If, in your previous "no cares about my weight" life, you would choose 6 different high-caloric food sources to eat while on vacation, limit this to 1. – *Anonymous*

50. If you are a busy mom and have trouble fitting in your exercise, try including your kids in your activities. Plan a trip to the park, go for a bike ride or play soccer with them. – *Anonymous*

51. If you are going to "treat" yourself to an obvious detrimental food source, ensure that it is a very high quality item, e.g. Godiva chocolate as opposed to a Three Musketeers Bar. – *Anonymous*

52. If you crave crunchy snacks as I do, prepare ahead and keep washed and cut veggies in the crisper. I recommend carrots, celery, radishes and cassava. – *Roshna K.*

53. If you get bored with water, get sparkling water and squeeze a lemon or lime for flavor. – *Celeste W.*

54. If you get tired and hungry around 3 p.m., like I do, drink a glass of ice water, eat a healthy snack and take a quick walk around the building. – *Anonymous*

55. If you have a craving for pizza, make a personal-sized pizza using a whole-wheat, low-carb tortilla, low-fat cheese, tomato sauce, chicken and lots of veggies! – *Anonymous*

56. If you have dinner plans at the home of friends/family who tend to eat unhealthy foods, offer to bring something healthy. – *Anonymous*

57. If you like things that are sweet, like chocolate, during Phase One, drink a sweet diet soda like Coke Zero. – *Celeste W.*

58. If you're a dessert person try Yoplait light yogurt (key lime pie, Boston cream pie, banana cream pie) as a dessert after dinner. – *Celeste W.*

59. Instead of butter on steamed veggies, use Italian herbs seasoning. – *Celeste W.*

60. If you get a craving, immediately drink a full glass of water and reach for the crunchy veggies! – *Anonymous*

61. Keep a food journal as well as a habit journal. – *Pam M.*

62. Keep a *good* food/exercise diary. – *Lanna F.*

63. Keep a picture of yourself, from when you were overweight, in various places such as a refrigerator door, vanity in your bathroom, etc. – *Anonymous*

64. Keep frozen veggies on hand for emergencies. – *Anonymous*

65. Keep healthy foods prepared and available; hard-boiled eggs from the fridge make a great protein snack. – *Joyce B.*

66. Leave the house if you have a craving. – *Carole H.*

67. Logging the food you eat on a website to track your progress is helpful. I recommend Sparkpeople.com; it has a huge food database. Also, drink the recommended amount of water per day! *– Marquel F.*

68. Make a batch of vegetable soup with whatever you have in your fridge. *– Anonymous*

69. Make a meal an "experience": light candles, soft music, etc. Do *not* eat "on the run." *– Anonymous*

70. Make a quick smoothie with low-fat yogurt, a handful of berries and ice cubes. *– Anonymous*

71. Make an extra serving of whatever you are preparing (chicken, fish, lean beef) for dinner to take and eat over salad for lunch the next day. *– Anonymous*

72. Make it easier on yourself by preparing your meals earlier in the week and reheating them. *– Anonymous*

73. Never eat dessert at a restaurant. *– Anonymous*

74. Pick a grocery day and stick to it. Then bring your groceries home and promptly clean and cut up your veggies for salads and snacks, grill some chicken and cut into strips to go over salads, boil some eggs, etc. A little preparation goes a long way! *– Anonymous*

75. Plan ahead for eating out by checking out the menu online. Many restaurants offer nutritional information online. *– Anonymous*

76. Put up an "old" picture and progress pictures as you lose weight. *– Lanna F.*

77. Put your fork down after every bite and do not pick the fork up again until all the food has been swallowed. – *Anonymous*

78. Remember to eat the proper amount of food exchanges according to your plan, on schedule, even if you aren't hungry. And drink your water! – *Joan B.*

79. Save your favorite snack for the end of the day so you have something to look forward to. – *Anonymous*

80. Schedule your workouts for the upcoming week and treat them as you would an important business meeting. – *Anonymous*

81. Share dishes at restaurants. So many restaurants provide huge portions. – *Anonymous*

82. Snacks! Don't skip your snacks. I lose less weight when I skip snacks because I tend to eat more during my main meals. Baby carrots for snacks are easy and convenient. – *Anonymous*

83. Stay away from fast-food places, even though they advertise "healthy" choices. There are few if any "good" choices. – *Anonymous*

84. Staying busy doesn't allow me to eat out of boredom. – *Samantha P.*

85. Sugar-free gelatin is a quick, healthy snack that is Phase One friendly. – *Anonymous*

86. Swimming is a great exercise: no pressure on your joints and you get a great and fun calorie-burning workout. – *Anonymous*

87. The trouble with water is that sometimes it can get boring. To jazz it up I offer the following tips. In the winter, boil water and add fresh lemon, or have a weak herbal tea (caffeine free) like mint, chamomile or ginger. Try white coffee, a drink offered in the Middle East as an alternative to the traditional Turkish coffee. It is a cup of boiled water with a few drops of orange blossom water (which can be purchased at a Near Eastern grocery store). It is refreshing, aids digestion and has a delightful scent (as does rosewater). *– Ina R.*

88. The three P's, Planning, Preparation, and Positive Thinking.... These will help you succeed. *– Anonymous*

89. Think of an activity like knitting to give your hands something to do while you watch a television show or movie. *– Anonymous*

90. Treat the gain of 3 pounds as urgently as you would treat the gain of 30. *– Anonymous*

91. Treat yourself to non-food treats and rewards, like a new book, movie or clothes. *– Rose A.*

92. Try pickled vegetables for a salty snack. *– Anonymous*

93. Use a smaller plate size for reducing portions easily. *– Lynn W.*

94. Use balsamic vinegar as a salad dressing because it tastes great and it's low in carbs. *– Anonymous*

95. Use banana peppers and hot pepper sauce to add flavor. *– Anonymous*

96. Weigh everything you eat. *– Lanna F.*

97. Weigh your food and keep strict control of your portions. – *Anonymous*

98. Weigh yourself once a week and keep a clipboard above the scale. Have defined parameters that will govern how you proceed from a dietary standpoint based on your weight. – *Anonymous*

99. When the weather is not cooperating with your outdoor cardio sessions, walk at the mall. Most malls are open at 7 a.m. for walkers, offering a safe, climate-controlled environment! – *Anonymous*

100. Write down everything that you eat, in a diary. – *Anonymous*

Your Own Pearls?

We hope you find these pearls appealing and useful, and we urge you to think of your own and write down those that have been most helpful for you. You will then have your own string of pearls to admire, if you find you are slipping back into old habits.

9. The Essential Guide to Eating on the Serotonin-Plus Weight Loss Program

By Julia K. Yuskavage, M.S., R.D.

Background

Our Transitional Diet Plan™ provides maximum, safe weight loss through a satisfying eating plan that you can stick to and, more importantly, want to stick to. The biggest complaint about the plan is that there is actually too much food! You will learn to fill up on lean proteins, vegetables, and low-fat dairy, while making healthy fruit and carbohydrates choices in moderation. A small amount of healthy fat tops it off.

We make it as easy as possible to lose weight while feeling good; we even provide a shopping list for every patient that details the foods to stock up on for each phase of the program. To begin a healthier lifestyle, you should eat a variety of healthy foods to obtain maximum nutrition. Focus on adequate lean protein with minimal saturated and trans-fat, plenty of non-starchy vegetables, moderately low-fat dairy, high-fiber fruits, complex carbohydrates and just enough healthy fats.

How Do Food Choices Influence Metabolism?

The food choices you make, as well as how you eat them, affect metabolism. Metabolic rate is based on several factors, including genetics, age, sex, physical activity level, muscle mass and food intake. We recommend eating 5 to 6 times throughout the day, including breakfast, lunch, dinner and 2 or 3 snacks. Doing so keeps your metabolic rate high during the day, meaning your body is working to burn calories all day long. Eating frequently during the day also prevents extreme hunger, which helps you avoid the after-work binge nine-to-fivers feel so often.

The Transitional Diet Plan is effective because it is based on choosing higher-protein, higher-fiber, lower-sugar foods. Again, we emphasize lean proteins to avoid excess fat and calories. Did you know that 3 ounces of trimmed, cooked lean meat provides about 200 calories? When choosing beef, look for words like round, loin or 90-95% lean ground beef. Lean cuts of pork include tenderloin, Canadian bacon, boneless ham 90-95% lean and leg shank.

You have probably heard that nuts are healthy. While they do contain protein and healthy fats, their high-fat nature warrants reserving them for when you have gotten closer to your weight loss goal. Our clinical experience is that nuts and peanut butter often hinder weight loss efforts. Therefore, they are not introduced until the later phases.

Read on to learn more about how each food choice can influence your weight.

Fats to Avoid. Avoid foods with high amounts of saturated fat, which are associated with greater risk of heart disease. These include certain oils (palm and palm kernel), high-fat animal-based products (butter, whole milk, full-fat cheese, sausage, bacon, hot dogs, marbled beef), desserts (cheesecake, ice cream, pies, doughnuts, cookies) and condiments (regular mayonnaise, sour cream, salad dressing).

Make a point to avoid trans-fat, which is more harmful than saturated fat and is associated with increased risk for heart disease, cancer and type 2 diabetes. You will find trans-fat in shortening, high-fat baked goods like doughnuts and cakes, frying fats, salty snacks (french fries, crackers and microwave popcorn) and some margarines. Many modern margarine and butter spreads now include small amounts of plant-based saturated fats (palm and palm kernel), which should be chosen instead of those made with trans-fat. Avoid trans-fat by shunning foods with the words "partially hydrogenated oil" or "shortening" in the ingredient lists.

Healthy Fats. Moderate use of unsaturated fats offers health benefits without a large amount of calories. Monounsaturated fat (found in olive oil, canola oil, avocados, nuts and seeds) lowers LDL cholesterol and triglycerides when it replaces dietary saturated fat. The consumption of polyunsaturated fat (found in high amounts in corn, safflower, soybean and sunflower oils) is associated with lower risk for heart disease, but it is important to consume the right balance of healthy fats. This means you should consume a higher ratio of omega-3 to omega-6 polyunsaturated fatty acids, since studies show that a higher intake of omega-6 fatty acids may cause harmful inflammation in the body. Food sources with high levels of omega-6 fats include soybean oil, corn oil, sunflower oil, safflower oil and cottonseed oil. An easy way to increase the balance of omega-3 fatty acids in your diet is to use primarily olive or canola oil, instead of those oils mentioned above. When eaten twice per week, fatty fish (salmon, trout, mackerel and tuna), flaxseed, walnuts and grass-fed beef provide omega-3 fatty acids, which decrease the risk of cardiovascular disease.

Fruits and Vegetables. Fruits and vegetables are integral to strong health and are recommended as part of the Transitional Diet Plan. Whole fruits and vegetables in their natural state offer fiber and plentiful nutrients, as well as antioxidants, which are molecules that prevent damage to cells. Deeply pigmented food such as blueberries, cherries, and carrots often contain the highest levels of antioxidants.

Phytochemicals, which are plant-derived compounds, also benefit human health by preventing the accumulation of fat deposits in arteries. Examples include plant sterols and stanols (found in small amounts in vegetable oils, nuts, grains, legumes, fruits and vegetables), flavonoids (in fruits, vegetables, nuts, seeds, green tea, onions, soy and wine) and sulfur-containing compounds found in garlic and onions. The saying, "An apple a day keeps the doctor away" is not far from the truth, but be sure to wash fruit well to remove pesticides. Apples are a great choice because they are high in fiber and lower in sugar. Fruits such as blackberries, strawberries, cantaloupe, oranges, grapefruits and honeydew melon are also lower-sugar fruit choices. However, bananas, pineapples, mangos, kiwis, grapes and dried fruits are higher in sugar and should be eaten less often.

Dairy. Another important component of any sound eating plan is low-fat dairy products, which provide calcium, Vitamin D, and other vitamins and minerals (Vitamin A, Vitamin B12, riboflavin, potassium, magnesium, zinc and phosphorus). You can obtain these nutrients by choosing skim milk, nonfat yogurt and low-fat cheese. One serving (1 ounce) of low-fat hard cheese contains 4-5 grams of fat, so limit this to 1-2 ounces per day. Cottage cheese naturally contains less fat than hard cheese, which makes it a great dairy choice. Some patients prefer to mix it with yogurt for a different flavor and texture.

Nonfat Greek yogurt is naturally higher in protein, and many people enjoy its thick, creamy texture. One serving of skim milk or plain, nonfat yogurt equals 1 cup (8 ounces).

Carbohydrates and Diet. While many factors affect the blood glucose response to food (including the type of carbohydrate, amount, fiber, processing, cooking and physiological glycemic status), it is important to monitor total intake of carbohydrates to control blood glucose. One way is by using the diabetic exchange system, which is taught as part of our program (see "Food Labels and Exchanges," below).

Restricting carbohydrate intake leads to the breakdown of glycogen (the stored form of carbohydrates) for energy. When glycogen is depleted, the body uses fat for fuel. Although in the early phases of the Transitional Diet Plan carbohydrates are restricted to approximately 20% (60 grams), the final phase provides about 45% (180 grams). Other low-carbohydrate diets may promote a large intake of fatty foods. However, we advise you eat lean protein and low-fat dairy, while using low-fat cooking methods, since a diet high in saturated fat is associated with an increased risk of coronary artery disease. A high protein intake is also beneficial to prevent loss of muscle mass, while promoting primarily fat loss. Additionally, the inclusion of "good" carbohydrates in the forms of milk, yogurt and carrots prevents fatigue, so you still have energy. You can see that carbohydrate intake is not completely limited. We even have patients with type 2 diabetes start on Phase One and feel fine, whereas it might be harder for them to adhere to a severely carbohydrate-restricted diet.

Types of Carbohydrates. Carbohydrates are classified as simple or complex, based on chemical structure. Simple carbohydrates contain only one or two sugar molecules. Monosaccharides contain one sugar molecule and include glucose, fructose (found in fruits, vegetables and honey) and galactose (found in milk). Disaccharides contain two sugar molecules and include sucrose (also known as table sugar), lactose (a milk sugar) and maltose. Simple sugars are found both in healthy foods (fruits, vegetables, milk) and in refined and processed foods (syrup, soda, candy).

Complex carbohydrates, or polysaccharides, contain many sugar molecules linked together in a chain, and include starch and fiber. They are found in fruits, vegetables, legumes and grains. The more sugar molecules that are linked together, the more complex the carbohydrate. Starchy foods include grains such as wheat, rice, barley, oats (and grain products like bread and pasta), as well as potatoes, corn, yams and beans. Non-starchy vegetables like asparagus and spinach consist of a higher fiber-to-starch ratio. Although fiber is not completely digestible by humans, it greatly benefits gastrointestinal health, including improved function and reduced risk of specific disease states. An abundance of non-starchy vegetables fulfills both nutrient and fiber needs. Try asparagus, broccoli, cauliflower, eggplant, cucumber, peppers, Brussels sprouts, celery, Swiss chard, spinach, mushrooms, zucchini and radishes to gain the benefits of fiber.

Make an effort to choose complex carbohydrates packed with fiber, instead of refined carbohydrates. Refined carbohydrates are foods such as white rice, white pasta, white bread and high-sugar cereals that have had fiber and nutrients stripped away during processing. These foods consist of "empty calories" and should be a minimal part of your diet. On the other hand, foods such as beans, brown rice and barley contain generous amounts of fiber and nutrients and are therefore healthier choices. When you consume these foods, the starch is digested slowly as the fiber passes through the digestive system. Not only does this promote a feeling of fullness, but it also benefits blood sugar stabilization by preventing rapid glucose absorption. This, in turn, can help prevent blood sugar spikes, which can leave you feeling extremely hungry.

According to the American Dietetic Association, up until the age of 50, women need 25 grams of fiber and men need 38 grams of fiber each day. After age 50, women need 21 grams and men need 30 grams per day. An increased intake of whole grains and fiber also helps reverse insulin resistance, which is a precursor to diabetes. Insulin resistance is controlled through weight management, which includes a healthy eating plan and exercise. Many of our patients who come to us with diabetes or pre-diabetes attain healthier levels of blood glucose by following our Transitional Diet Plan and reducing dietary sugars.

Beverage Intake. Our patients always feel better and are more successful on the program when properly hydrated. As a general rule, we recommend drinking at least 8 glasses of water (64 ounces) per day. The Institute of Medicine recommends that sedentary persons drink 3.7 liters (125 ounces) of fluid daily, for men, and 2.7 liters (91 ounces) for women. You may enjoy artificially sweetened beverages (diet sodas or flavored waters) in moderation, but your cell metabolism works best with pure water. Humans are composed of approximately 60% water, so it is no wonder that many patients are most successful on the program when drinking pure water rather than artificially sweetened beverages. Another benefit of drinking adequate water is that is provides satiety, which helps you avoid eating too much. Water is essential for cell function, metabolic reactions, digestion and absorption of food and excretion.

Limit caffeinated beverages to 1 or 2 per day, since caffeine is a diuretic and is dehydrating. We recommend that you drink one extra cup of water for every cup of caffeinated beverage you consume. Drink enough water throughout the day so that your urine is a pale yellow color. Experiment with decaffeinated herbal teas to increase your fluid intake; there are many delicious flavors available.

Although alcohol provides some health benefits when consumed in moderation, we recommend avoiding all alcohol in the beginning of the Transitional Diet Plan, since it is a source of empty calories, interferes with normal metabolism and contributes to dehydration. Alcohol has almost as many calories per gram as fat (7 in alcohol versus 9 in fat). In fact, fat metabolism is basically put on hold when you drink alcohol, in order to metabolize the alcohol first. Additionally, excessive alcohol consumption often leads to mindless eating. After several weeks on the plan, you may choose to drink a light beer or white wine spritzer on occasion.

What Will You Eat?

To give you an idea of one day's menu on our Transitional Diet Plan after Phase One, you might start with an egg, vegetable and turkey omelet for breakfast, followed by a midmorning snack of raw vegetable strips and low-fat cottage cheese. Lunch might be a hearty portion of grilled shrimp, steamed cauliflower and a handful of fresh berries. Your mid-afternoon snack could include nonfat-fruited yogurt or kefir (a yogurt drink that aids digestion) with a medium-sized orange, while dinner could be a large serving of grilled flank steak, plentiful vegetables and a side salad with light salad dressing.

Sounds like a lot of food, right? In fact, most of our patients tell us that there is too much food to eat and they don't feel hungry. The only difference for Phase One would be the exclusion of fruit and increased protein servings.

We encourage snacks such as fresh vegetables, sugar-free gelatin and low-fat dairy or protein sources. For example, you might make an egg salad using several hard-boiled eggs, Dijon mustard and celery. Dip fresh vegetables in a tablespoon of hummus, roll up some turkey around pepper strips, or enjoy a light flavored yogurt. These snacks not only prevent hunger throughout the day, but also keep your metabolic rate higher.

Dining Out. Our staff offers support 100% along the way, whether you need advice for an upcoming dinner out or even selecting portion sizes. Loading up on a large salad topped with grilled chicken is always a safe choice. Order a low-fat dressing, such as vinaigrette, on the side so you can control how much you use. Or, simply use a drizzle of olive oil and vinegar. Try to choose fresh steamed vegetables as side dishes, instead of starches (potatoes, rice, pasta). When you do choose a starch, make it high-fiber and whole-grain rather than re-fined. For example, brown rice and whole-wheat pasta are high-fiber options. Order all sides without butter, and do not accept the bread or chip basket. Avoiding cream sauces saves calories; look for low-calorie condiments such as salsa and mustard rather than mayonnaise, ketchup (which is higher in sugar) and special sauces.

Before an outing, eat a healthy snack that you know fits in with your dietary plan. Choose one that combines lean protein and fiber (such as half an apple with 1 ounce of low-fat cheese), so you feel full and satisfied. Sharing an entrée at restaurants is acceptable, and it usually provides plenty of food for two people. If you have an absolute favorite dish, search for the nutrition information online or in the restaurant so you know exactly what is in it. Choose water, diet sodas or unsweetened tea to avoid calories from beverages.

Portion Sizes. It is no surprise that portion sizes have grown over the years, so it is important to recognize how much food you need for sustenance and not eat beyond that point. The size of your palm, or the size of a deck of playing cards, is about 3 ounces of cooked meat. One ounce of cheese looks the size of a 9-volt battery, and ½ cup of vegetables is about the size of a tennis ball. These portion sizes are often larger when we dine out.

We recommend investing in a food scale, which typically costs under $10, to weigh cooked ounces of meat, poultry and fish. Once you do this for one or two weeks, you will soon be able to estimate the weight just by looking at the portion size.

Filling up on non-starchy vegetables is a good method for appetite control. Generally, 1-2 cups of a raw vegetable is an appropriate portion to have with a meal. Consume fruit in amounts similar to the size of your cupped hand. This may be 1 cup of fresh berries, ½ medium banana or a medium-sized apple. Our staff recommends eating fruits, rather than drinking them, due to the concentrated sugars in fruit juices, which contribute to excess calories and can quickly spike blood sugar. If you must have fruit juice, limit your serving to 4-6 ounces a few times a week. The same goes for dried fruits, which are dense in sugars. A serving of dried fruit should only be about 2-4 tablespoons.

Food Labels and Exchanges. Reading food labels is another important skill you will learn in our program. According to the diabetic exchange list, 15 grams of carbohydrates equals 1 carbohydrate exchange. As an example, you may be told to eat 2 carbohydrate exchanges each day at a particular phase of the

Transitional Diet Plan. Using the diabetic exchange standard above, one carbohydrate exchange is equal to 1 slice of bread, ⅓ cup cooked rice, ½ cup cooked oatmeal and so on. We provide you with a complete list of common carbohydrate exchanges. You can also calculate the number of carbohydrate exchanges for a particular item by reading the nutrition facts label.

Suppose you want to know how many carbohydrate exchanges are in your favorite brand of cracker. First, look at the total grams of carbohydrates. Let's say that 1 *serving* of the cracker contains 18 total grams of carbohydrates. Second, look at the total grams of fiber. If your favorite cracker contains less than 5 grams of fiber per serving then you need not go any further. You know that 1 serving of your favorite cracker is equal to little over 1 carbohydrate exchange, using the 15 grams of carbohydrate = 1 carbohydrate exchange guideline.

However, if your favorite cracker contains 5 *or more* grams of fiber per serving, then according to the 2008 American Diabetic Association guidelines you can subtract *half* of the fiber from the total grams of carbohydrates to calculate the "net" carbohydrates per serving. This is because your body does not break down all of the fiber you ingest, and it simply passes through your digestive system. Suppose your favorite cracker is now available in a high-fiber option that includes 6 grams of fiber. You would subtract 3 grams of fiber (half of 6) from the total carbohydrates (18 grams) and your net carbohydrates equal 15 grams. Therefore, the high-fiber option of your favorite cracker is a better choice because it is equal to (not greater than) 1 carbohydrate exchange. Plus, it gives you the health benefits of fiber.

Be sure to note the serving size when reading the nutrition facts label. If the label lists 8 crackers as 1 serving size, providing 15 grams of carbohydrates, and you eat 16 crackers, you know you ate not just 1, but 2 carbohydrate exchanges, for a total of 30 grams of carbohydrates.

Vegetarianism. Vegetarians can thrive on our program, despite the emphasis on adequate protein. Tofu is a versatile, high-protein food and can be enjoyable when you get creative. A soybean curd, tofu contains fiber, healthy fat, plentiful nutrients and about 10 grams of protein per 4 ounces. Several convenient vegetarian options include Boca Burgers or Garden Burgers and other similar products found in most grocery stores. You can even purée tofu with vegetables for soups, blend it with fruit for a smoothie, or mash it into sandwich spreads, season it as dips or sauté it in a stir-fry.

Depending on individual limitations, foods such as cheese, milk, yogurt, fish, seafood, poultry and eggs may be protein choices in the vegetarian diet. Zinc, Vitamin D, Vitamin B12 and iron are found in high amounts in animal products, so a daily multivitamin containing these nutrients may be necessary for some vegetarians. A multivitamin is provided to all patients on the Transitional Diet Plan.

Conclusion

We are confident that our comprehensive guidance will assist you in your weight loss goals. Reaching a healthy weight is important, but it is equally important to maintain that weight over time. Losing weight takes commitment by learning and adhering to healthier eating behaviors. While the success rate of our patients is very high when they follow our program, we understand that each person is unique and different. Therefore, we work with you to overcome problems or difficulties you may have while on the program. Most times, a little tweaking here and there is all it takes to fit individual needs.

From choosing healthier foods to finding your motivation for becoming healthy, our clinicians are here to help!

10. Recipes for Success

By Julia K. Yuskavage, M.S., R.D.

Beginning on the following page are 20 recipes that will take you from breakfast to dinner, morning to evening, and fit nicely into the Transitional Diet Plan. They taste good and will fill you up, while providing excellent nutrition. The number of food group exchanges is listed for each dish. I hope you enjoy preparing healthy dishes for yourself and your family as much as I do! *Bon appétit!*

Turkey Meatloaf

Makes 8 servings
Serving size: 1/8 of the loaf
Ingredients
- 2 pounds 98% fat-free ground turkey
- ½ cup skim milk
- 1 cup Italian breadcrumbs
- 1 tablespoon dried oregano
- 2 large eggs, beaten
- ½ cup chopped onion
- ½ cup chopped green pepper
- 1 cup grated carrot
- ¼ cup ketchup
- 1, 8-ounce can tomato sauce
- Salt and black pepper to taste

Directions: Preheat oven to 400 degrees F. In a large bowl, mix all ingredients except green pepper and tomato sauce, until well combined. Coat a baking dish with cooking spray and transfer mixture to the dish. Shape meat into a loaf. Spread tomato sauce and green pepper over meatloaf. Cook for 1 hour or until a thermometer inserted in the center reads 170 degrees F. Remove from oven. Cool for 10 minutes before serving.

Exchanges per serving: 4 protein, 1 carbohydrate. (The 15 grams of carbohydrates in this recipe comes from ingredients such as ketchup and breadcrumbs.)

Beef Pot Roast

Makes 6 servings
Serving size: 4 ounces beef topped with ½ cup mushrooms
Ingredients
- 6 cups fresh mushrooms, chopped
- ½ cup chopped onion
- 1 ¾ pounds beef chuck roast, boneless
- 1 cube beef bouillon
- 2 cups hot water
- ½ teaspoon fresh rosemary, chopped
- Black pepper to taste

Directions: Coat a large saucepan with cooking spray. Add mushrooms and onions. Cook until onions are tender. Add the roast to the saucepan and cook until brown on all sides. In a medium bowl, combine beef bouillon cube with hot water; stir until dissolved. Add rosemary and pepper to beef broth. Pour over roast. Cover and simmer over low heat, about 2 hours or until roast is tender. Slice and serve.

Exchanges per serving: 4 protein, 1 vegetable

Seafood Stew

Makes 4 servings
Serving size: approx. 1.5 cups
Ingredients
- 3 garlic cloves, minced
- 1 tablespoon grated lemon peel
- 1 ½ cups low-sodium vegetable broth
- 1, 15-ounce can tomatoes, drained and diced
- 1 bay leaf
- ¼ teaspoon crushed red pepper flakes
- 3 tablespoons fresh parsley, chopped
- Salt and black pepper to taste
- 2, 6.5-ounce cans clams with juice
- 1 pound skinless snapper fillets, cut into bite-sized pieces
- ½ pound fresh or frozen scallops

Directions: Coat a large saucepan with cooking spray. Cook garlic and lemon peel over medium heat, for 3-5 minutes. Add broth, tomatoes, bay leaf, red pepper flakes, parsley, salt and pepper. Bring to a boil and cook for about 10 minutes. Add clams, snapper and scallops. Cover and simmer about 10 minutes or until fish flakes with fork and scallops are opaque. Serve seafood mixture in 4 bowls; spoon broth on top.

Exchanges per serving: 9 protein, 0.5 vegetable

Veal with Mixed Vegetables

Makes 4 servings
Serving size: approx. 1 cup
Ingredients
- 1 teaspoon olive oil
- 2 tablespoons lemon juice
- 3 garlic cloves, minced
- 2 tablespoons fresh parsley, chopped
- 4 sprigs fresh thyme
- 1 ¼ pounds veal cutlets, cut into strips
- ½ cup diced red onion
- ½ cup diced celery
- 2 cups fresh mushrooms, chopped
- 1 cup cherry tomatoes, chopped

Directions: In a large bowl, combine olive oil, lemon juice, garlic and herbs. Place veal strips in mixture, toss to coat, and let marinate 15 minutes in refrigerator. Coat a large skillet with cooking spray and add onion, celery, mushrooms, tomatoes and veal. Cook until vegetables are tender and veal strips are browned. Serve immediately.

Exchanges per serving: 4 protein, 1 vegetable

Baked Crab Cakes

Makes 4 servings
Serving size: 2 cakes
Ingredients
- ½ cup diced red bell pepper
- ½ cup diced green bell pepper
- 1 ¼ pounds crab meat
- 1 large egg, beaten
- 1 tablespoon lemon juice
- 1 teaspoon Worcestershire sauce
- 1 tablespoon light mayonnaise
- 1 tablespoon Dijon mustard
- 2 teaspoons seafood seasoning
- Black pepper to taste
- ¼ cup Italian bread crumbs

Directions: Preheat oven to 350 degrees F. In a medium skillet, heat cooking spray and sauté bell peppers until tender. Remove any shell from crabmeat. In a large bowl, whisk together egg, lemon juice, Worcestershire sauce, mayonnaise, mustard, seafood seasoning and black pepper. Gently mix in crabmeat, bread crumbs and cooked peppers. Shape mixture into 8 cakes and place on baking sheet coated with cooking spray. Bake until cakes are golden brown on each side (about 20 minutes), flipping cakes over once during cooking. Serve immediately.

Exchanges per serving: 4 protein, <0.5 vegetable, <0.5 carbohydrates, <0.5 fat

Grilled Pork Kabobs

Makes 4 servings
Serving size: 2 kabobs
Ingredients
- 1, 14-ounce can vegetable broth
- 2 garlic cloves, minced
- 1 tablespoon dried oregano
- 1 tablespoon dried thyme
- 1 ¼ pounds lean pork loin, cut into bite sized cubes
- 1 cup fresh mushrooms
- 1 large red onion, cut into wedges
- 1 large red bell pepper, cut into squares
- 1 large green bell pepper, cut into squares

Directions: In a large bowl, mix together broth, garlic, oregano, thyme. Add pork cubes, mushrooms, onion, red pepper and green pepper to bowl and mix to combine. Marinate overnight in refrigerator. Remove pork and vegetables and arrange pork on 8 skewers, alternating with mushrooms, onions and peppers. Grill for about 25 minutes or until done, turning the skewers halfway through cooking. Slide pork and vegetables off skewers and serve.

Exchanges per serving: 4 protein, 1 vegetable

Pan Roasted Beef Tenderloin

Makes 6 servings
Serving size: approx. 5 ounces
Ingredients
- ¼ cup balsamic vinegar
- 2 garlic cloves, minced
- 1 ½ teaspoons dried rosemary
- 1 ½ teaspoons dried thyme
- 1 teaspoon extra virgin olive oil
- ½ teaspoon whole black peppercorns
- ½ teaspoon black pepper
- 2 ¼ pounds beef tenderloin

Directions: Preheat oven to 425 degrees F. In a small bowl, mix balsamic vinegar, garlic, rosemary, thyme, oil, whole peppercorns and pepper together. Rub the mixture into the beef. Place the tenderloin fat side up on the rack in roasting pan. Tuck small "tail" under the rest of the loin so the thin end of the roast becomes thicker and cooks more evenly. Tie at 3-inch intervals with kitchen string. Place on a rack in roasting pan. Place meat thermometer in thickest section of beef. Roast at 425 degrees F for 40-50 minutes or until thermometer reads 150 degrees F minimum. Remove from oven and cover beef tightly with foil. Let stand, covered with foil, for 15 minutes. Remove string and meat thermometer; carve beef and serve.

Exchanges per serving: 5 protein

Curried Lamb

Makes 4 servings
Serving size: approx. 1 cup lamb, ½ cup cooked rice
Ingredients
- 1 ¼ pounds lean lamb, trimmed of fat and cubed
- ½ cup diced white onion
- 2 garlic cloves, minced
- 1 cinnamon stick
- 1 cup beef broth
- 2 teaspoons curry powder
- ½ teaspoon salt
- ½ teaspoon black pepper
- ¼ teaspoon ground ginger
- ½ teaspoon turmeric
- 1 teaspoon cumin
- 2 cups chopped tomato
- 1 cup chopped green bell pepper
- 1 tablespoon all-purpose flour
- ½ cup grated carrot
- 2 cups brown rice, cooked

Directions: Heat cooking spray in a large saucepan over medium heat. Add lamb and sauté for about 5 minutes, turning until brown. Add onion, garlic and cinnamon to the saucepan. Sauté until onion is clear. Then, stir in broth, curry powder, salt, pepper, ginger, turmeric, cumin, tomato, green pepper and flour. Mix well. Cover, reduce heat, and simmer about 40 minutes, or until the lamb is tender. Stir occasionally. Mix grated carrot with brown rice and serve ½ cup rice per bowl. Serve even portions of lamb and vegetables over rice.

Exchanges per serving: 4 protein, 1 vegetable, 1 carbohydrate

Pork with Apples

Makes 4 servings
Serving size: approx. 4 ounces pork, ½ cup apple mixture
Ingredients
- 1 ¼ pounds pork tenderloin, trimmed of fat
- ¾ teaspoon salt
- teaspoon black pepper
- 1 tablespoon fresh rosemary, chopped
- 1 tablespoon fresh thyme, chopped
- ½ cup chopped white onion
- large Granny Smith apples, chopped
- garlic cloves, flattened
- 1 cup low-sodium beef broth

Directions: Preheat oven to 450 degrees F. Season pork tenderloin with salt, pepper, rosemary and thyme. Heat cooking spray over medium heat in a saucepan large enough to hold tenderloin. Add pork and sear on all sides until brown (about 5 minutes). Remove pork from saucepan and place in a baking dish. Add onion, apples and garlic to saucepan and heat until golden (about 5 minutes); add to the baking dish, surrounding pork. Roast for about 15 minutes or until thermometer inserted in the center reads 160 degrees F. Apples should be soft. Remove pork, transfer to plate and let stand for 5 minutes. Then, pour broth over apple mixture in saucepan previously used. Stir over high heat for about 2 minutes. Cut pork diagonally and serve topped with apple mixture.

Exchanges per serving: 4 protein, 1 fruit

Vegetarian Chili

Makes 6 servings
Serving size: approx. 1.5 cups
Ingredients
- 1 teaspoon vegetable oil
- 22 ounces extra firm tofu, drained and crumbled
- 1 cup chopped mushrooms
- ½ cup diced white onion
- ½ cup diced green bell pepper
- 3 garlic cloves, minced
- ½ teaspoon cumin
- 3 tablespoons chili powder
- 2 bay leaves
- 1, 14-ounce can tomato sauce
- 1, 28-ounce can diced tomatoes, with liquid
- 1, 28-ounce can white kidney beans, drained and rinsed

Directions: In a large pot, heat vegetable oil and sauté tofu over medium heat for 3 minutes. Add mushrooms, onions, peppers, garlic, cumin, chili powder and bay leaves. Cook until vegetables are tender (about 5 minutes). Add tomato sauce, tomatoes and beans. Bring to a boil, reduce heat, cover and simmer about 50 minutes. Remove bay leaves prior to serving.

Exchanges per serving: 3 protein, 1 carbohydrate, 1.5 vegetable

Salmon Patties

Makes 4 servings
Serving size: 2 patties
Ingredients
- 20 ounces salmon, canned
- 1 tablespoon Dijon mustard
- ¼ cup Italian bread crumbs
- 2 tablespoons fresh parsley, chopped
- 1 large egg, beaten
- ½ cup finely chopped red onion
- ½ cup chopped celery
- ½ teaspoon paprika

Directions: Mix all ingredients in a medium bowl. Divide and shape mixture into 8 patties. Coat skillet with cooking spray, turn to medium heat, and heat patties until golden brown. Serve immediately.

Exchanges per serving: 4 protein, <0.5 carbohydrate, <0.5 vegetable

Beef Stir-Fry

Makes 4 servings
Serving size: approx. 4 ounces beef, ½ cup vegetables
Ingredients
- 2 garlic cloves, minced
- 1 tablespoon fresh ginger, peeled and minced
- 1 large onion, sliced
- 1 ¼ pound beef tenderloin, thinly sliced
- 1 cup broccoli florets
- 1 cup red pepper, chopped
- 1 cup fresh mushrooms, sliced
- 1 teaspoon Dijon mustard
- Black pepper to taste

Directions: Heat cooking spray in a large skillet over medium heat. Cook garlic, ginger and onion until softened. Add beef tenderloin and cook until lightly browned. Add broccoli, red pepper and mushrooms. Cover and cook for 5 minutes, stirring. Mix in mustard and pepper. Cover and cook for 5 minutes, stirring. Remove from heat and mix before serving.

Exchanges per serving: 4 protein, 1 vegetable

Crust-less Quiche

Makes 6 servings
Serving size: 1/6 of the quiche
Ingredients
- ½ cup chopped white onion
- 2 cups chopped fresh asparagus
- 2 cups sliced fresh mushrooms
- 1, 10-ounce package frozen chopped spinach, thawed and drained
- 6 large eggs, beaten
- 1 lb skinless, boneless chicken, cooked and shredded
- 6 ounces shredded low-fat mozzarella cheese
- ½ cup salsa
- Salt and black pepper to taste

Directions: Preheat oven to 350 degrees F. Coat a 9-inch pie pan with cooking spray. Then, coat a skillet with cooking spray and heat over medium heat. Add onions, asparagus, mushrooms and spinach. Cook until excess water evaporates from spinach. In a large bowl, combine eggs, chicken, cheese, salsa, salt and pepper. Add vegetable mixture and mix to combine. Pour mixture into prepared pie pan. Bake for about 45 minutes or until eggs are set. Cut into 6 even slices and serve.

Exchanges per serving: 4 protein, 1 vegetable

Citrus Thyme Chicken

Makes 4 servings
Serving size: ½ chicken breast, ½ orange
Ingredients

- 2, ½-pound skinless, boneless chicken breasts (halved)
- Salt and black pepper to taste
- 2 large oranges, thinly sliced
- ½ medium red onion, chopped
- 2 tablespoons fresh thyme, chopped
- 3 garlic cloves, minced
- ¼ cup balsamic vinegar

Directions: Preheat oven to 375 degrees F. Coat a baking dish with cooking spray. Season chicken breasts with salt and pepper. Arrange chicken breasts in one layer in baking dish and spread orange slices evenly over chicken. Add onion, thyme, garlic and balsamic vinegar. Bake for 20 minutes or until chicken is opaque inside and juices run clear when cut in the middle. Serve immediately.

Exchanges per serving: 3 protein, 1 fruit

Savory Pumpkin Soup

Makes 4 servings
Serving size: approx. 1 cup
Ingredients
- 1 teaspoon vegetable oil
- 2 tablespoons diced white onion
- 2 cups canned pumpkin
- 1 cup low-sodium chicken broth
- 1 packet chicken bouillon (approx. 3.5 grams)
- 1 cup skim milk
- ½ teaspoon nutmeg
- 1 teaspoon dried parsley
- Black pepper to taste

Directions: In a medium saucepan, heat vegetable oil and sauté onion for 3-5 minutes, until onion turns clear. Add remaining ingredients and whisk thoroughly. Cook over medium heat for 10-15 minutes, stirring occasionally. Serve immediately.

Exchanges per serving: 1 carbohydrate, <0.5 milk

Vegetable Chicken Stew

Makes 6 servings
Serving size: approx. 1.5 cups
Ingredients
- ½ medium white onion, chopped
- 3 garlic cloves, minced
- 1 ¾ pound skinless, boneless chicken breasts, thawed and cubed
- 4 cups low-sodium chicken broth
- 1 cup cold water
- 2 cups chopped celery
- 2 cups chopped Swiss chard
- 3 small potatoes
- 1 ½ cups canned garbanzo beans
- 2 cups chopped mushrooms
- 1 tablespoon cornstarch
- 1 teaspoon cumin
- 1 teaspoon chili powder

Directions: Coat a large saucepan with cooking spray. Cook onions and garlic for 3-5 minutes, until onions are clear. Set aside. In same saucepan, add chicken cubes and cook until slightly browned. Add chicken broth, water, celery, Swiss chard, potatoes, garbanzo beans and mushrooms to the saucepan. Transfer ¼ cup broth to a small bowl; add cornstarch bit by bit, whisking to mix so lumps do not appear. Slowly pour mixture into large sauce to thicken broth, whisking. Add cumin and chili powder. Bring to boil. Reduce heat to low; cover. Simmer for 20 minutes. Remove from heat. Let cool before serving.

Exchanges per serving: 4 protein, 1 vegetable, 1 carbohydrate

Hearty Breakfast Oatmeal

Makes 2 servings
Serving size: approx. ½ cup cooked
Ingredients
- ½ cup dry old-fashioned oats
- 1 egg white
- 2 cups skim milk
- 1 teaspoon cinnamon
- 1 teaspoon vanilla extract
- 1-2 packets Splenda
- 2 cups fresh berries
- 2 tablespoons slivered almonds

Directions: Stir to coat oats with egg white in a medium bowl. Add oats and milk to medium saucepan. Turn heat to medium and stir. Cook oatmeal, stirring occasionally, until oatmeal thickens. Remove from heat. Add cinnamon, vanilla and Splenda. Serve 1 cup of oatmeal in each bowl. Add 1 cup of berries and 1 tablespoon of almonds to each bowl. Serve immediately.

Exchanges per serving: 1 carbohydrate, 1 milk, 1 fruit

Cauliflower Mash

Makes 2 servings
Serving size: approx. ½ cup
Ingredients
- 2 cups chopped cauliflower
- ½ cup cold water
- ¼ cup skim milk
- ½ teaspoon garlic powder
- Salt and black pepper to taste
- 2 ounces shredded low-fat cheddar cheese

Directions: Place 2 inches of water and chopped cauliflower in a medium saucepan and steam until fork tender. Drain residual water. Mash the cauliflower until it reaches potato-like consistency, adding in skim milk. Season with garlic powder, salt and pepper. Garnish each serving with ¼ cup low-fat cheddar cheese.

Exchanges per serving: 1 protein (cheese may also be counted as 1 milk), 1 vegetable

Cabbage Rolls

Makes 5 servings
Serving size: 2 rolls
Ingredients
Sauce:
- 1 teaspoon olive oil
- 1 cup chopped white onion
- 2 garlic cloves, minced
- 1, 28-ounce can peeled tomatoes with juice
- 1 cup canned tomato sauce
- ½ teaspoon salt
- ¼ teaspoon black pepper
- 14 large green cabbage leaves

Filling:
- 1 ¼ pounds ground round beef
- ½ cup minced white onion
- 1 garlic clove, minced
- 1 tablespoon dried dill weed
- 2 tablespoons fresh parsley, chopped
- 2 large eggs, beaten
- 3 tablespoons ketchup
- ¼ cup dry old-fashioned oats

Directions: Preheat oven to 400 degrees F. To prepare sauce, sauté onion and garlic in oil in large saucepan until onion turns clear. Stir tomatoes with juice and canned tomato sauce into pan. Add salt and pepper. Cover pot with lid, keep heat on low and simmer for 20 minutes. Set aside. Bring a pot of water to a boil and place cabbages leaves in boiling water for 3 minutes. Remove leaves and place in colander under cold running water.

Mix all filling ingredients in large bowl. Make 10 cabbage rolls. To assemble rolls, place about ¼ cup filling in each leaf. Fold sides and bottom of leaves to enclose mixture. Repeat until filling is used up. Line pan with 4 leaves. Place leaves, seam side down, on pan. Pour sauce over rolls. Cover with foil. Bake for 45 minutes or until thermometer inserted in a cabbage roll reads 180 degrees F. Let cabbage rolls cool for several minutes and serve.

Exchanges per serving: 4 protein, 1.5 vegetable, <0.5 carbohydrate

Baked Tofu with Zucchini

Makes 4 servings
Serving size: approx. 4 ounces tofu, ½ cup zucchini
Ingredients
- 18 ounces firm tofu
- 4 cups thinly sliced zucchinis
- 3 tablespoons soy sauce
- 3 tablespoons balsamic vinegar
- 3 garlic cloves, minced
- Salt and black pepper to taste

Directions: Preheat oven to 375 degrees F. Drain water off tofu. To drain remaining moisture, wrap tofu in paper towels and place heavy skillet on top for 20 minutes. Chop tofu into bite sized pieces. Toss tofu and zucchini cubes with soy sauce, balsamic vinegar, garlic, salt and pepper. Let marinate in the refrigerator for 45 minutes. Coat baking pan with cooking spray and arrange tofu and zucchini on pan. Bake for 10-15 minutes on each side, or until edges of tofu start to brown. Remove zucchini when browned on edges. Serve immediately.

Exchanges per serving: 4 protein, 1 vegetable

11. Exercise and Weight Loss

By Donna L. Eckenrode, MPAS, PA-C

Background

Exercise means different things to different people. For some, it has a positive connotation and is a regular activity that they look forward to. For many, it is a necessary evil, but tolerable. For others, exercise stirs up feelings of dread and fear. Yes, fear! For someone who is overweight, the thought of getting into exercise gear and going to the gym or even walking in the neighborhood is intimidating. In addition, it is uncomfortable to perform normal daily activities, let alone exercise, when you are carrying around extra weight.

I know what you're thinking: "What does she know about being overweight?" Actually, a lot! When I delivered my daughter, I weighed 185 pounds, which is heavy for my barely 5′2″ stature. I managed to gain 55 pounds during my pregnancy, so I know how it feels to institute an exercise program as an overweight female. I have learned a great deal about exercise through my education and research, but I have also learned a lot during my own journey, and most of all from talking with my patients. I hope that by sharing my thoughts I can ease some of your anxiety and perhaps even change your perspective about exercise.

But first, a disclaimer and a plea: consult a physician before starting an exercise program to ensure that you are healthy enough for physical exertion.

Why Exercise?

Regular exercise is often praised as the panacea for a number of medical problems. Studies have shown that outcomes for several diseases, including cardiovascular disease, thromboembolic stroke, hypertension, type 2 diabetes, osteoporosis, colon cancer, breast cancer, anxiety and depression improve with regular physical activity. All of these conditions have a direct correlation with obesity, in that your risk of developing them increases if you are overweight or obese. Many patients who enter our weight loss program shed or reduce their blood pressure-lowering, cholesterol and diabetic medications by the end of their 12-week program. I cannot guarantee that weight loss and regular exercise will allow you to discontinue medications, since there are also genetic forces at play, but these conditions will improve to some degree with weight loss and regular exercise. This is particularly true for those individuals with type 2 diabetes.

Diabetes. The increasing prevalence of excess weight and obesity has led to an unprecedented epidemic of type 2 diabetes, and is likely to be followed by an epidemic of patients with complications from it. For years, diet and exercise have been the cornerstone of treatment. In fact, the guidelines of the American Diabetes Association recommend that an individual with type 2 diabetes perform at least 150 minutes of moderate intensity aerobic exercise or at least 90 minutes of vigorous aerobic exercise per week. Aerobic exercise improves glucose control, enhances insulin sensitivity and reduces cardiovascular risk factors, including a reduction in adipose tissue (fat) around the internal organs, improved lipid profiles and improved arterial function.

Glucose (sugar) levels in the blood decline with exercise due to the improvement of glucose uptake by the tissues and skeletal muscles resulting from decreased insulin resistance. Insulin is a chemical that is released from the pancreas in response to the presence of glucose in the bloodstream. The body's tissues, including skeletal muscle and the liver, respond to the presence of insulin and take up sugar from the bloodstream. However, in a patient with type 2 diabetes, the body's tissues become desensitized to the presence of insulin and fail to transport glucose from the bloodstream efficiently, which is known as insulin resistance.

When exercise is combined with diet to promote weight loss, the improvement in metabolic control is greater than that seen with exercise alone. I have observed patients with type 2 diabetes who are participating in the Serotonin-Plus Weight Loss Program discontinue their use of insulin or reduce their oral medications within a matter of weeks due to the combination of diet and exercise. If you consider the long-term effects of diabetes, which include increased risk of heart attack and stroke, kidney disease or failure, loss of sensation or pain in the extremities and impaired or loss of vision, the positive effects of diet and exercise in the treatment and prevention of diabetes are profound.

Hypertension. Many of my patients are diabetic, and most of them are hypertensive. Hypertension is a disease that is literally near and dear to my heart, because I am a sufferer myself. I was diagnosed with high blood pressure in my mid-20s and continue to require medications despite being the healthiest I have ever been. I am an example of the profound implication that genetics can have on an individual's health, since my maternal grandmother and two of my aunts suffered with high blood pressure as young adults.

However, I am in the minority. The association between obesity and hypertension is strong, irrespective of age, race and gender, and the risk of hypertension increases proportionally with weight. Research has shown that an 8 kg (17.6 pound) weight loss decreases blood pressure from 122/81 mm Hg to 110/74 mm Hg (deviation of +/-2 mm Hg) in normotensive obese patients and 149/98 mm Hg to 135/86 mm Hg (deviation +/-3 mm Hg) in hypertensive obese patients. This translates to an average 12-14 mm Hg decline in systolic blood pressure and a 7-12 mm Hg drop in diastolic pressure. I have seen similar results in patients enrolled in the Serotonin-Plus Weight Loss program.

Moderate aerobic exercise has been shown to lower blood pressure. When you look at the long-term effects of hypertension, which include increased risk of heart attack, stroke and kidney disease, the benefits of regular exercise and weight management are significant. Overall, exercise has a favorable effect on cardiovascular risk factors, specifically on the reduction of hypertension, hyperlipidemia (high cholesterol), obesity and blood lipid profiles. High cholesterol is associated with plaque build-up in the arteries, a condition referred to as atherosclerosis, which can lead to heart attack and stroke.

Mood. You have heard that individuals who exercise lead happier and longer lives. Research has shown that exercise has positive effects on psychological behavior and can help in the improvement of general mood.

Getting Started

Now that you know the multiple benefits of weight loss and regular exercise, let's work up a sweat. Since you will be more likely to do an activity that you enjoy, do your best to make exercise fun! Why torture yourself doing what your friend or neighbor does for exercise? You can choose from many activities, most of which you can perform to some degree at every fitness level. Here are some ideas:

1. Walk. Get a good pair of shoes and find a place to walk, such as your neighborhood, the mall, an indoor or outdoor track, a park, a treadmill or even your living room.

2. Run. Get a good pair of running shoes and a good venue.

3. Swim. You can do water aerobics or simply swim, walk or run laps in the pool.

4. Bike. You can do this outdoors on an upright or recumbent bicycle, or indoors on a stationary machine. Spinning classes are great, too.

5. Dance. You can choose from many fun and easy-to-do workout videos and classes that involve dancing. Or turn on your radio or favorite CD at home and just dance to the music. I love to do this with my daughter.

6. Do aerobics. "Aerobics" can be intimidating to many people. When I hear the word I think of Jane Fonda in a leotard and leg warmers in one of her videos from the 1980s. There is an entire industry of workout videos and classes that include aerobics—dance, step, boxing, yoga, weight training or a mixture of these—to help with your weight loss efforts.

7. Do activities with your children. Kids have a lot of energy, which can be quite contagious. Take your children to the playground or the local pool, play ball with them, or walk, bike, run or dance with your kids.

8. Play interactive video games. These are the latest in video game technology and the greatest because they encourage children to be more active. They appeal to adults as well

because they are fun and can be done by individuals of varying fitness levels. Many of my patients and family members use the interactive video systems as part of their exercise regimen, which includes aerobics, strength training, yoga and balance exercises. When my family gets together for the holidays, we now play the Wii instead of traditional board games.

Once you know what you want to do for exercise, you need to put it into action. The greatest challenge is finding the time, in our very busy lives, which may involve juggling the demands of work and home. The key is to *make* time. If you fail to take the time to exercise and get healthy now, you may not be around to work or spend time with your spouse or children later.

Try to exercise consistently on the weekends, giving you at least 2 days a week of activity. This way you only have to worry about getting another 2-3 days during the busy workweek. Pick a time that works best for you. If you are a morning person, do your workouts in the morning before work. However, if you are like me and can't imagine functioning before 7 a.m., schedule your workouts for later. You may also want to exercise during your lunch hour. Many companies are trying to promote better health practices among their employees by offering on-site gyms. If you have this resource, take advantage of it by working out during lunch or before going home. If your company does not have a gym, you can still go for a brisk walk outside or even indoors if your work environment has long hallways.

If you belong to a gym, go straight to the gym before going home. Once you get home, you are more likely to get distracted and may lose your motivation to get back in your car to drive to the gym. If you prefer to exercise at home, do so in a room away from the common areas, where there is likely to be more hustle and bustle. You will be better able to focus on your workout, free from distractions.

If you have young children, as I do, it is difficult to make free time. You might try to schedule your exercise sessions after the kids go to bed or before they wake up in the morning. Another alternative is to invest in a sturdy stroller or running stroller for walking or running, while your child enjoys the ride.

The American Heart Association recommends that adults engage in 30 minutes of "moderate-intensity" aerobic exercise five days a week, or "vigorous-intensity" aerobic activity for a minimum of 20 minutes three days a week. Moderate-intensity exercise is equivalent to a brisk walk that noticeably accelerates the heart rate, and vigorous-intensity exercise is an activity that causes rapid breathing and a substantial increase in heart rate. In addition, adults should perform activities that maintain or increase muscular strength and endurance, a minimum of two days each week. Specifically, 8-10 exercises using the major muscles of the body should be performed on two or more non-consecutive days each week.

These recommendations can seem overwhelming if you are just starting an exercise program. We often set our exercise goals too high by saying, "I'm going to work out for 30 minutes five times this week." Wednesday rolls around and we haven't done anything. We feel defeated and say, "Well, maybe next week will be a good time to start my exercise routine." In order to avoid this common pitfall, I ask my new patients to set a reasonable goal of 2 sessions of exercise, for 15-20 minutes each, during the first week of our program. If you can do more when starting an exercise regimen, do so.

As each week goes by you should increase your exercise, either by expanding the amount of time you exercise per session or the number of sessions per week, until you at least meet the recommendation given above. If you are already exercising 5 days a week, keep up the good work and try challenging yourself with interval training or re-sistance/strength training sessions (discussed below).

Maximizing Your Workouts

Whether you are a busy parent, working long hours, going to school or a combination of all the above, finding the time for exercise can be very difficult. Unlike celebrities, we do not have the luxury of spending 2-3 hours daily in the gym, so it is important to maximize your workouts. Two good ways to do this are strength training and high-intensity interval training. I recommend you do a little of each.

Strength Training and Aerobics. I would like to provide you with some background information in regards to the science behind exercise. Maximal aerobic power, referred to as aerobic capaci-ty, or VO2 max, measures the rate at which you can expend energy during exercise. It is used to discuss an individual's exercise performance, particularly for study purposes. While some athletes may take the time to calculate their predicted VO2 max or actually have it measured with exercise testing, most of us have no reason or desire to do so. A better way to measure your exercise performance or intensity is by calculat-ing and using your target heart rate, which I will discuss in greater detail below.

As we age, our VO2 max declines. In fact, the formula to calculate predicted VO2 max involves the subtraction of your age. The decline in exercise capacity with aging contributes to weight gain. In order to counteract this decline and perform the same level of total energy expenditure (or calories burned) during exercise, an individual may require an increase in the amount of exercise time overall as they age. Hence, we need to do regular aerobic exercise, and more of it, to help maintain our exercise capacity with aging. Further complicating the picture, skeletal muscle or lean muscle mass, which is an important determinant of resting metabolic rate (or "metabolism"), also declines with aging. Strength training exercises are therefore necessary to counteract the loss of muscle mass associated with normal aging.

Research has shown that strength training and aerobic exercise each significantly improve performance and exercise capacity in obese women, meaning an individual's capacity to expend energy ("burn" calories) during exercise improves with regular aerobic and strength training types of exercise. While both forms of exercise increase VO2 max, aerobic exercise is more effective according to a study comparing aerobic and strength training exercises in the absence of a dietary program.

Aerobic and strength training exercises are each helpful, but the combination of both is ideal in maximizing your weight loss or weight maintenance efforts. The best way to get the most out of your limited exercise time is by combining the two with circuit training, during which resistance-training exercises are interspersed with aerobic activity. Recent studies have shown that circuit training performed three times a week, in combination with healthy eating behaviors, stimulates the greatest weight loss and improvements in measures of body composition, such as waist circumference.

Interval Training. Another way to maximize your workouts is through high-intensity interval training. Interval training can be done with almost any cardiovascular exercise. "Interval" can refer to *an interval* of distance or time, though most individuals will measure time while performing intervals. In simple terms, to perform high-intensity interval training (HIIT) you need to perform more vigorous exercise for an interval of time or distance before returning to a lower-intensity or recovery pace. Then repeat, and repeat and repeat. You can vary the intensity by changing the speed or resistance, or both. An example of HIIT would be to jog for 4 minutes, run for 2 minutes, return to jogging and repeat this pattern for 20-30 minutes. I recommend that you do a 5-minute warm-up and cool-down to avoid injury.

If you're a walker you don't need to jog; you can perform HIIT by walking as fast as you can for 2 minutes, then at a lower-intensity or recovery pace for 4 minutes and then repeat. I am using the 2 to 4 minute ratio as an example. While the ratio for high-intensity to lower-intensity exercise should be 1:2 or 1:4 depending on your level of fitness, the length of the intervals can be manipulated. For example, you can do intervals of 30 seconds of high-intensity exercise followed by 1 minute of lower-intensity exercise (1:2), or 30 seconds of high-intensity exercise followed by 2 minutes of recovery (1:4). If you were to do intervals using distances as a measurement, you would run for ¼ mile, jog for ½ mile and repeat. A great place to perform distance intervals is on a local track, where you can do lap intervals (jog 2 laps and run 1 lap or jog the straight-aways and run the curves).

You can do HIIT with activities like walking, running, swimming or biking. In general, your recovery or lower-intensity exercise should be paced so it is relatively easy to hold a normal conversation, and the higher-intensity intervals should correspond with an ability to speak but not hold a normal conversation.

If you are a little more numbers-oriented, the best way to track intensity when doing intervals is by measuring your heart rate, or pulse. As mentioned earlier you can use your target heart rate as a measure of your exercise intensity. Your target heart rate is determined by subtracting your age from 220. The high-intensity intervals should be done at 80-95% of your target heart rate, while the recovery or lower-intensity portions should be 40-60%. For a 31-year-old, like me, the higher-intensity heart rate would be a pulse of 150-180 beats per minute (0.95 x [220-31]), while the rate for the lower-intensity or recovery periods would be 100-113 (0.6 x [220-31]).

HIIT has been shown to be safe and well tolerated in patients with a variety of cardiopulmonary diseases, including chronic obstructive pulmonary disease and congestive heart failure, and even patients who have had coronary-artery bypass surgery or a heart transplant. Nevertheless, you should tailor your interval training to a pace that is suitable to your level of fitness.

HIIT maximizes your workouts for several reasons. First, it burns more total fat than sustained exercise at a lower intensity, since overall more "work," or energy, is expended per workout. By working at short durations of high-intensity, you can burn more calories overall. However, the benefits do not stop there. Research has shown that what happens after exercise, not only during exercise, makes a difference. Exercise increases your metabolism for a while after completion of the exercise. The "catch-up effect" the body has in response to exercise is referred to as EPOC, or excess post-exercise oxygen consumption, and can last as long as 48 hours following intense cardiovascular exercise. To understand why, think of this. When you climb a set of stairs, when do you breathe the hardest? Not until you reach the top, right? The same phenomenon occurs after high-intensity exercise, resulting in increased metabolism, or EPOC.

Research has proven that anaerobic exercise, including strength training and HIIT, is associated with the largest increases in EPOC. In addition, remember that VO2 max tends to decline with aging and contributes to weight gain. Studies have shown that after 6 weeks of HIIT, untrained individuals raised their whole body VO2 max, thus increasing the ability to achieve greater levels of oxygen consumption during exercise, and thus burn more calories.

Now that you are more knowledgeable on HIIT and strength training, you can get started on making the most of your exercise routines.

Thoughts on Walking

Though I am a runner, I am a big advocate of walking for exercise. Most of us have been walking our entire lives, so there is nothing to learn, and it is inexpensive and can be done in a variety of settings. All you need is a decent pair of shoes and a sidewalk, mall, treadmill, track or your living room. If you walk at home, there is no pressure or stress about having to work out in front of others, which can be intimidating if you are overweight or obese. You can purchase DVD programs that guide you through a walking routine in the comfort of your own home.

Even people with physical limitations can usually walk for exercise. While the intensity may vary between individuals, any movement that increases your heart rate is going to be beneficial and provide a starting point for your exercise regimen. When I started walking for exercise after the birth of my daughter, I weighed about 170 pounds and felt fatigued after 20-30 minutes of brisk walking while pushing the stroller.

Depending on the weather and my energy levels as a new mother, I would walk 3-4 times a week for 20-30 minutes. After a few weeks, I began to lose weight and found pushing the stroller at a brisk pace for 30 minutes was easier, so I began to walk longer and more days a week. Before I knew it, I was walking 45-60 minutes daily with the stroller and doing light resistance training 2-3 times a week. Once I "maxed out" the intensity at which I could walk, I started jogging and then running. I still walk frequently for exercise as a cross-training or recovery activity.

The point is that walking is an exercise that most individuals can perform in starting and maintaining an exercise regimen. As with any exercise, you need to gradually increase the amount you do until you are exercising at least 5 days a week for 30 minutes.

Running

I am addicted to running! The funniest thing about *me* running is that I used to hate it. I never minded sprinting because I am petite with short, strong legs, but long-distance running was never my forte, in high school or college. In fact, I volunteered to be the goaltender for my lacrosse team in college because I would rather have hard rubber balls hurled at me than run. I really *hated* running! So how did I go from that to my current addiction to running? Here's my story.

My Journey. After the birth of my daughter, once I had maxed out my walking and transitioned into jogging (as discussed above), I got a running stroller from a co-worker, and I gradually increased my intervals until I was running exclusively.

I decided to set a goal for myself. I entered a local 4-mile race, desiring only to finish. I met my goal and had a little extra energy at the end for a sprint. I finished at a 10-minute-per-mile pace and felt great. I decided to up the ante a little further and trained for a 10k (6.2 miles) race, which was just a month after the 4-miler. The 10k went well and I was able to maintain my 10-minute/mile pace without difficulty, followed by completing a half-marathon (13.1 miles) at a 9:47 per mile pace only 5 months after my first race.

Recently, I was in Virginia Beach for the Shamrock Marathon, which I completed in 5 hours and 18 minutes. Though I was slowed by a bruised heel, I reached the finish line and ended my run with a "strong" finish. I still find it hard to believe that *I* ran 26.2 miles at a 12-minute pace, which is not bad for a first marathon. Nine months had passed between my first race and my first marathon, and while training to run a marathon is not the same as being pregnant, during my natural-birthing classes, the instructor would often compare preparing for labor to training for a marathon. In my case, it was a good analogy.

I offer this sketch of my journey to give you a perspective of where I am coming from as the writer of this chapter. In addition, it provides an example of how you can continue to challenge yourself in order to stay on track with your exercise regimen.

If You Want to Run. While I now enjoy running, I do not expect all my patients to share my enthusiasm. In fact, I do not recommend running as an exercise regimen for anyone who is obese. The excess weight places a lot of stress on the joints, particularly the knees. By the time I initiated jogging/running as a part of my exercise regimen, I weighed 135-140 pounds, meaning I was overweight but not obese for my height.

If you are interested in running for exercise, you should introduce it gradually, as intervals, once you find fast walking is no longer difficult. You can gradually increase your running intervals, then transition to runs of 1-2 miles in duration and work your way up from there.

There are some general rules of thumb if you are going to run for exercise. Invest in a good pair of running shoes. Many running stores perform free gait/stride evaluations and can recommend a shoe that is best for you. By using a proper-fitting shoe that is appropriate for your stride, you are less likely to experience ailments and injuries (shin splints, bruised heels, stress fractures, iliotibial band syndrome) that can plague runners. In general, you should replace your running shoes every 500 miles, which depending on your weekly mileage can be every 6 weeks to every 6 months.

This brings me to my next point: you should keep track of your weekly mileage. Not only does this allow you to know when to buy new shoes, but it will help you set goals. To prevent injury you should avoid increasing your mileage greater than 10 % from the previous week. For example, if you start by running 2 miles a day, 5 days a week, for a total of 10 miles a week, you should not run more than 11 miles (10% of 10 miles is one mile and 10+1=11 miles) the following week. This gives your body time to adjust to the stress from running, through improved muscle tone and blood flow, which helps prevent injury.

Another good practice is to vary the surfaces you run on. I quickly discovered that I could not run on concrete and black-top surfaces consistently without experiencing injury. Concrete is the hardest of all the surfaces and, in turn, hardest on your joints. Running on blacktop is a better alternative, though still not ideal. Dirt or cinder trails are the best surfaces because they offer less impact on the joints. I try to run a dirt or mulch trail at least twice a week and do a speed or interval workout once a week at the local track. I do the rest of my runs usually on blacktop with the occasional stretch of concrete sidewalks.

Take a day off from running to rest or do a cross-training activity such as swimming, biking or aerobics. Listen to your body. If you experience pain that persists for more than a few minutes, stop running and stretch and restart once the pain subsides. If the pain returns with activity or persists while at rest or walking, you may need to see a physician.

Stretching

Regular stretching can improve circulation, range of motion, posture, joint stiffness, muscle tension and your ability to relax. If you have ever taken yoga, which involves breathing and stretching in a variety of poses, you can attest to the benefits of stretching. I see stretching as a necessary evil, but I have found that a little bit goes a long way. Unfortunately, the recommendations for stretching are conflicting. While my coaches always focused on pre-game stretches, research suggests that stretching before exercise does not prevent injury. Post-workout stretching or stretching after warming up has been suggested to be most beneficial. I recommend that you only stretch warmed-up muscles. Take a light walk for several minutes while gently moving your arms, then ease into each stretch for the first 15 seconds by stretching to the point where you feel mild tension on the muscle. Once the tension eases, go a little farther until the tension increases again. To avoid injury, do not bounce! The stretch should not be painful; if it is then back off. Hold your stretches for at least 30 seconds, and up to 60 seconds for a really tight muscle. Remember to breathe.

Conclusion

Whichever exercise you choose—running, walking, swimming, biking—continually challenge yourself and make your workouts fun. By going a different route, trying a new aerobic video or class or dusting off your bike and taking it for a spin, you will prevent boredom and keep your body guessing. Plan your exercise routine one whole week at a time.

Remember that your exercise routine is just that, *your* exercise routine. You should try to view it as the time you make for yourself each day, or at least 5 times a week. My exercise time has been a great way for me to relieve stress. I frequently find myself thinking about work and home situations while I'm out for a run, often with greater clarity than usual, or planning my activities for later in the day. By taking time out for myself, I find I have more quality time with my daughter and husband, free of mental distractions.

Patients tell me that they feel guilty about taking time away from their spouse, children and work to exercise, and I must admit that as a mother of a young child I often feel the same way. But think of it this way: if you fail to exercise and maintain a healthy weight and lifestyle now, your time with loved ones may be less overall. It makes me happy to think that I will have the opportunity to be with my daughter when she gets married and has children of her own. These thoughts often keep me going during my runs and keep me on track with my health maintenance.

12. Maintaining a Healthy Weight and Lifestyle

By Donna L. Eckenrode, MPAS-PA-C

Background

Staying at a healthy weight is as important as attaining it. There are thousands of diet books and programs that help you lose weight, but not many that tell you how to keep it off. Unfortunately, there is no magic bullet to maintaining your weight loss; if there were, all those celebrities who yo-yo up and down in their weight would have used it to their advantage.

Maintenance is often more difficult than weight loss. The sacrifices you have made and the exercise you have done religiously over the past months need to be continued. Overall, the short-term changes you have instituted to lose the weight now need to become long-term, lifestyle modifications. That is the secret to maintenance. Now that you know this, you will never have to diet again, right? You can go about your business and simply continue what you have been doing for the last several months for the remainder of your days. My job is to provide you with insight and perhaps even inspiration to help you maintain your weight loss indefinitely so you will never have to diet again.

It Requires a Change in Your Thinking

As a physician assistant at Serotonin-Plus Weight Loss I have come to understand that the problem with maintaining a healthy weight is our *thinking*. I was conducting a final visit with a patient who had lost 60 pounds on our program, when she said to me, "It's sort of depressing, knowing that I can never eat like I did before." At that moment, I realized that not only do I, as a practitioner, need to try to help my patients with their behaviors (eating right and exercising), but I need to try to alter their thinking. I gently told my patient that she needs to continue to exercise regularly, follow the nutritional recommendations we had impressed upon her during her program and continue to take her Serotonin-Plus supplement to control carbohydrate cravings.

More importantly, I tried to change her perception of what makes her happy, not "depressed" (the word she used), by reminding her how great she feels when she looks in the mirror and sees a healthy individual; when she puts on a pair of jeans that hasn't fit in years, or when she meets with a friend she hasn't seen in awhile and is greeted with, "You look fabulous!" I challenged her to find happiness with her new activities and body, such as setting and achieving her exercise goals, wearing a smaller size and feeling more comfortable and confident in social situations. Then I asked her to think about how good she feels at her current healthy weight versus how she felt when she was 60 pounds heavier. I urged her to remember how poorly she felt then as compared to now, especially when she feels tempted to eat unhealthily or to slack off in her exercise regimen. By the end of our discussion, she was refocused and re-energized in regards to maintaining a healthy weight and lifestyle. I don't think I changed her perception or thinking in just one visit, but I provided her with positive items to focus on when she feels depressed or overwhelmed.

The point is that maintaining a healthy weight and lifestyle requires changes be made in regards to your thought processes.

Putting Theory into Action

Now that you know why maintenance is so difficult, the question is, how do you make it easier? As you have probably discovered, it requires thought to be healthy, whereas it requires little or no thought to eat poorly and to be inactive. It is very easy to pick up dinner at a fast-food restaurant after a busy day. On the contrary, it takes thought and planning to have something healthy available in the refrigerator once you get home. Likewise, it takes planning to pack workout clothes so you can stop at the gym after leaving work. I stress the importance of planning and preparation to my patients at every visit, and Dr. Posner often gives similar advice in his blog, which I encourage my patients (and you) to read daily.

Eating Real Food. To be healthy and maintain a normal weight, you must eat *real* food. That's why programs like Nutrisystem don't work long-term, resulting in weight regain once the program is over and the dieter is done eating the pre-packaged foods. If you have to eat real food, you have to prepare real food. How do you find the time to prepare healthy meals amid the hustle and bustle of our busy lives?

If you guessed thoughtful planning and preparation, you guessed right. Designate one day (many people choose Sunday) as your grocery day, so that every week you can get the items needed for the remainder of the week. Then, plan your meals for the upcoming week and buy the appropriate items for those meals and snacks. This way, you are not left stranded wondering what to make for lunch or dinner, and you will not run out of healthy snacks during the busy work week. Once you get back from the grocery store, clean and cut vegetables for snacks and salads and place them into containers so that you can grab them quickly when needed. If I know it will be a particularly busy week for me, I will grill some chicken breasts or lean hamburger ahead of time and place them in the refrigerator for later in the week.

If you don't mind leftovers, you can cook an extra portion or two of your evening meal for meals later in the week. I find this to be very helpful, especially since I work evenings twice a week. I cook on Sunday, Tuesday, Thursday and Saturday, while the leftovers cover the remaining days. If you decide not to use the leftovers for the next night's dinner, you can always pack the leftover protein in your lunch for the next day. I have found, as have my patients, that a little bit of planning and preparation early in the week goes a long way to maintaining a healthy lifestyle.

Plan for Exercise. Likewise, you need to plan your exercise regimen. By planning ahead, I do not mean you have to write down your plans for the week. I am not one to write things down, but if you find that writing your weekly goals and plans is helpful, please do so. What works for one person does not and will not necessarily work for another.

On that note, look at your schedule for the upcoming week and, if applicable, your spouse's and children's schedules. Based on the activities planned for the week, decide which days you can and cannot exercise. For example, I have an office meeting scheduled for Thursday evening, so I know at the beginning of my week that I will need to work out Thursday morning before work or use Thursday as a rest day. In addition, if I have an appointment to schedule, like a visit to the dentist, I will try to schedule it for my rest day so it will not interfere with my weekly exercise schedule.

While your goal should be to exercise 5 days a week for at least 30 minutes, life will get in the way occasionally and 5 days a week will be impossible. However, since something is better than nothing, always make your best effort to exercise some time during the week. If you expect to have a particularly challenging week in regards to exercise, make sure you are even more diligent in adhering to your diet. You may want to reduce your daily carbohydrate and/or fruit exchanges and increase your protein during a busier week, since you will not be able to exercise as regularly.

Set Goals. One of the keys to staying on track with exercise and maintaining a healthy weight is to set goals. If you are constantly working toward a personal goal, you have incentive to maintain your weight and will be more likely to hold yourself accountable. I set goals for myself with races. My first goal was to run a half-marathon, then to run and finish a marathon and now to run a marathon at a 10-minute-per-mile pace or less. Your personal goals may be less exercise-oriented, such as fitting into a pair of jeans or a little black dress you haven't worn in several years. Maybe your goal is to be a size 8 for your high school reunion or to wear a bikini this summer. These are great goals to keep yourself on track and your weight in check. However, you must set a new goal once you have reached your old one, so that you do not slip back into your old habits. Again, setting personal goals involves thinking and planning ahead.

Know Your Weight. To stay on track with your weight loss and maintenance efforts you need to be aware of your weight. It never ceases to amaze me the number of patients that come in for their first visit and are unaware of their actual weight. I have discussed this issue with patients, and it boils down to the fact that they simply do not want to know the truth. Avoiding the scale enables them to evade the reality that they are overweight or obese. I recommend you have a scale in your home and weigh yourself once a week. By performing a weekly weigh-in at home, just as we do with our patients in the office, you make yourself accountable for your weight. I tell patients that if their weight increases by 5 pounds, they should come back for a visit to get refocused. Remember, it is much easier to shed 5 pounds versus 15 or more.

Stay Active. Another important part of maintaining a healthy weight is to stay active. Being active is different from intentional exercise. Now that you are at a healthier weight, you will likely feel more comfortable in your body and less fatigued. I sit much less than I used to, due, in part to the fact I am chasing a toddler around my house. However, I am also frequently doing housework, such as vacuuming, mopping the floors, cleaning the bathrooms or running laundry up and down the stairs. I tend to walk places more frequently and consciously park further away from the storefront or take the stairs to get a little extra activity in every day. By spending more time moving and less time sitting, you will find it easier to maintain a healthy weight, get more things accomplished on your "to-do" list, feel more energetic and likely sleep better at night.

Take the Serotonin-Plus Supplement. Finally, continue taking the Serotonin-Plus Weight Loss Formulation and/or the Serotonin Plus multivitamin to control carbohydrate cravings. While you have already learned to eat smaller portions throughout the day to help control your appetite, those pesky carbohydrate cravings will still occur, particularly if you are feeling stressed. Since stress is usually present to some degree throughout our lives, taking a Serotonin-Plus supplement (either the multi-vitamin or weight loss formulation) will help prevent detrimental eating behaviors.

Managing Common Pitfalls

We all encounter common pitfalls in our weight loss and weight-maintenance efforts, but we can manage them well through thought and planning. Pitfalls for our patients (and me) include but are not limited to eating out, business travel/vacations and family gatherings/parties.

Eating Out. This is first on my list because it is probably the most common and most avoidable. We Americans are eating out more than ever, despite the downturn in the economy. In fact, according to statistics from the National Restaurant Association, 133 million Americans dine out every day, and the typical adult eats at a restaurant six times a week. There are a number of reasons why we dine out more than we used to, but basically, we eat out more often due to time constraints. It takes time to prepare a meal for yourself, let alone a family of four. This is where planning ahead comes into play. However, sometimes you have to grab something on the go, or you just need a break from meal preparation and would like to have a nice evening out with your family or friends. So how do you manage eating out?

First of all, try to pick a restaurant that has healthier options. If you are considering fast-food restaurants, opt for the made-to-order deli versus the burger joint, especially if the deli offers salads. If you want to go out for a nice dinner, avoid the all-you-can-eat buffet or the Italian restaurant with huge portions.

I like to go to restaurants that offer a variety of healthy salads and protein/meat selections.

Now that you have decided on a healthier venue for dinner, what are some things to avoid when ordering? In the fast-food setting, order grilled chicken or fish and lose the bun or opt for a salad. However, with fast-food salads the dressing is usually loaded with calories, so you may go without, order the dressing on the side and use it sparingly or use your own low-calorie dressing. Also, you want to opt out of the fries and choose a small baked potato (plain or with salsa), side salad with low-calorie dressing or fresh fruit instead.

At a sit-down restaurant, consider splitting an entrée with your spouse or friend, or plan to eat half and take the other half home for later. Avoid over-eating by drinking a lot of water or other no-calorie drink, not ordering an appetizer, dessert or alcohol, and skipping the bread or chips basket. When ordering protein options, such as steak, chicken and fish, avoid heavy sauces by asking the server to not brush, prepare or top your meat selection with butter, heavy sauces or excessive amounts of cheese. The same goes for vegetables.

Watch out for those salads. You think that by ordering a salad you are making a good decision, right? Not always true! Restaurants tend to top salads with fatty cheeses, croutons, bacon and heavy dressings. Carefully review what comes on a salad, and ask that the undesirables be left in the kitchen; order a low-fat or low-calorie dressing on the side. If you know where you will be going to dine, you might want to do some research ahead of time. Many restaurants offer nutritional information on their websites, so you can make a well-informed healthy decision ahead of time.

Travel. Whether for business or vacation, travel is problematic for individuals trying to lose weight or maintain a healthy weight. The biggest issue is that it usually involves a significant change in your daily routine. You may have to get up earlier or later than usual, which will change your meal and snack times. You can easily adjust your meal/snack times by simply eating every 3-4 hours.

You certainly need to plan your meals. If you are staying in a hotel or at a resort, call ahead and find out what meals they offer and what restaurants are in the area. When booking a hotel, consider one that offers a complimentary hot breakfast, which will enable you to start the day off right with eggs or a bowl of oatmeal and a glass of skim milk. For lunch, you can never go wrong by eating a salad with grilled protein, such as chicken or fish, which you can get at a local restaurant or even through hotel room service. Dinner should be limited to a vegetable and protein, and skip the dessert and alcohol.

What about snacks? Your hotel room may not be equipped with a refrigerator to keep items cool. However, you can call ahead and request a portable refrigerator for your room to keep bottled water and snacks, such as low-fat yogurt and cheese sticks, which you can pick up at a local grocery store or even pack to take with you in a cooler if you are driving to your destination. If a local grocery store will not be available and you are unable to pack a cooler, you can take some low-fat, low-carbohydrate protein bars to use for snacks. If your hotel provides a breakfast buffet, take a piece of fresh fruit back to your room for a snack later in the day. If you will be staying with friends or family, call ahead to find out what your host has planned for meals. You may even offer to prepare dinner one evening, which your host will likely appreciate.

You can also plan ahead in regards to exercise. If you will be staying at a hotel, try to book one with a pool or workout facility, and be sure to make time to get to the gym regularly. If you will be staying with family, ask if they have equipment you can use or if their neighborhood is good for taking a walk or run. I know you are thinking, "If I'm on vacation, do I need to go to the gym?" The answer to that question is no, but you need to do something to be active. You might walk a lot while sightseeing or decide to go for a swim or bike ride with your kids. Any of these activities, if done with intention and not at a leisurely pace, can count as exercise. However, if you want to have a glass of wine or indulge in a small piece of dessert as part of your vacation experience, remember in order to do this without derailing your weight loss and maintenance efforts you must make an extra effort to exercise.

Family and Other Gatherings. Another common pitfall is attending family functions and happy hours. There are some great strategies I have developed and learned from my patients that are helpful in avoiding unnecessary temptations at such events. First, if you think healthy snacks are likely to be scarce, you can volunteer to bring a vegetable tray or other healthy dish. If you are unable or it is inappropriate to bring a food item, as is the case with happy hour, eat something healthy before the event and snack lightly on high-protein or vegetable appetizers. Do not stand or sit near the food and dessert tables to avoid mindless or unnecessary eating. Drink water frequently in order to avoid overeating or indulging in high-calorie foods and drinks. You may want to take your favorite bottled water with you. If you are going to a happy hour, you can always order a club soda (no alcohol or calories) with lime or opt for a white wine spritzer (about 60 calories and equivalent to a serving of fruit). Avoid food or drink "pushers" and learn to politely say "No thank you."

Remember, you are in control of the situation. When temptations arise, ask yourself, "How will I feel about eating [fill in the blank] when I step on the scale at my weekly weigh-in?"

Or, "How many miles will I have to run to burn off this [fill in the blank] I just ate or drank?" These questions will help you maintain control over temptations and ultimately your weight.

Conclusion

As you can see, there are many strategies you can use to avoid sabotaging your weight loss efforts, despite attending events that are notoriously associated with high-calorie foods and drinks. I encourage patients, in preparing for an upcoming event that will be problematic, to make a list of things that may sabotage or slow down their efforts. Once they identify potential temptations, they can develop strategies to overcome each, and perhaps pick one allowable temptation during the event. For example, the last time I went home for Christmas I decided that I would allow myself one sample of my mother's famous blackberry pie. After I reviewed my mental checklist for Christmas day, I decided to forego wine with dinner and skipped the mashed potatoes. In addition, I tried to squeeze in a little activity that evening by playing an interactive video game with my family.

Not only does your body change when you lose weight, but your thought processes need to change as well. While indulging in a glass of red wine might once have been a way for you to relieve stress after a busy day, you may now find you are running to the gym or doing yoga at home in the evenings. Managing your weight and staying healthy is about changing your perception as to what makes you happy. Examine the new you versus the old you by making a list of your old thoughts and behaviors versus your new ones. Consider which of your new thoughts and behaviors make you feel good or happy, and try to focus on these positive points daily. I have found happiness in running and cooking, which were activities that I previously hated. The things that may have invoked negative feelings when you were overweight and unhealthy may now be tolerable and even enjoyable.

While your weight loss journey may be over, in the words of the Carpenters, "We've Only Just Begun" your weight maintenance. Maintaining a healthy weight and lifestyle involves a daily commitment that requires thought and planning. It is very easy to lose focus and slip back into old habits, so every day I ask myself, and encourage you to do the same, "What am I going to do today to be healthy?" If you find yourself slipping back into your old ways and need a gentle push in the right direction, be sure to give us a call at Serotonin-Plus Weight Loss (and maintenance!) so we can help you refocus and reenergize your efforts.

13. Serotonin-Plus Patient Testimonials

Compiled by Julia K. Yuskavage, M.S., R.D.

There is no greater form of advertisement than word of mouth. It is truly priceless! More importantly, when we decided to put this publication together, we at Serotonin-Plus Weight Loss agreed that we wanted to give our patients an opportunity to be heard. We have asked some of our most successful patients to share their individual weight loss journeys and Serotonin-Plus Weight Loss experiences, in hopes their stories and advice will inspire and aid you in your own weight loss and maintenance efforts.

Sue Hillmer
55-year-old Caucasian female

To be honest, my number-one reason for losing weight was to look better. However, I knew that by losing the weight, my health would improve, too. What finally got me to do it was deciding with my husband to take this journey together and then visiting Dr. Posner for a consultation for the Serotonin Plus Weight Loss Program to see if it would "fit" our lifestyle.

This was not my first attempt at weight loss. When I was in my teens and living at home, my mother and I joined TOPS (Take Off Pounds Sensibly), and I lost a few pounds but nothing memorable. In my mid-20s, I went on the Scarsdale Diet and, again, I lost some weight but nothing memorable. When I was in my mid-30s, I joined Jenny Craig and lost 50 pounds. I looked great and felt great but got too comfortable in my current weight and lost sight of my ultimate weight loss goal. Eventually, I gained back all of the weight, and then some.

I have always believed that any diet, no matter how good or bad for you, will "work" as long as you stay on it. The minute you stop following the diet, you gain back the weight. The key is changing your lifestyle, and that is what I did on the Serotonin-Plus Weight Loss Program. Strangely, I thought the hardest part of being on the program would be eating out. However, the most difficult hurdle for me was satisfying my sweet tooth. I overcame this by opting for healthy alternatives. Discovering sugar-free gelatin and sugar-free popsicles, as recommended by Dr. Posner, kept my sugar intake low. They are extremely low in calories and yummy!

The first two weeks of the program were hard for me to adjust to, as I was eating new foods and more protein than usual. But overall, I felt great during the first 12 weeks. Once I lost the first 5-10 pounds, I felt like I was on a roll and didn't want to do anything to sabotage myself. I also continued my workout sessions with a personal trainer twice a week. On weekends, my husband and I would bike with our cycling group, riding 20-30 miles each Sunday.

I actually reduced my cholesterol and blood pressure medication over the course of my weight loss. When my husband and I began the Serotonin-Plus Weight Loss Program, we were both on medication for high blood pressure and high cholesterol. Within three months' time, we were able to stop taking this medication and have stayed off ever since. My husband was supportive, especially since he was on the plan. In addition, I had support from my personal trainer. I lost 65 pounds total, 50 pounds of which was lost in just under 6 months.

Some of the most helpful parts of the program were the support of Dr. Posner and his staff at weekly weigh-ins, the daily blog that Dr. Posner wrote, and accountability. His blog was helpful, encouraging, interesting and sometimes even humorous. I knew that Dr. Posner was invested in our weight loss just as we were, and I felt comfortable in knowing that he would not let us fail. Regarding accountability, the weekly weigh-ins encouraged us to stick with it and maintain healthy eating. Trying to do this "on my own" would not have worked for me. The accountability of the weekly weigh-in visits was a primary motivating factor in keeping me focused, and as a result I realized weekly weight losses throughout the program.

From my personal success, I learned that eating a nutritious breakfast high in protein keeps you satiated longer than a high carbohydrate breakfast. I always keep nutritious snacks on hand. I really thought that I would be hungry based on the daily calorie intake prescribed by the program. However, the appetite suppressant and serotonin supplement helped curb my hunger. As I lost weight, my energy levels increased. The second phase of the program filled my need for carbohydrates and fruit, and provided many food choices. I can honestly say that I never felt hungry in all the time I was on the program. When I got closer to my goal weight, my mantra was portion control. For example, I did not deprive myself of any of the traditional holiday foods, but I did exercise proper portion control by placing a "sampling" of each dish on my plate. In this way, I never felt like I was doing without and still got to enjoy the foods I like.

I will have kept the weight off for a year, come July 2010. What has helped keep the weight off is that I continue to exercise as I did while on the program and also continue to eat the same way as I did on the program. My husband and I learned a new way of eating, have incorporated that into our lifestyle and have not fallen back into our old eating habits.

My best advice for others is that before you begin the program, get rid of all the junk food in the house and any other foods/drinks that will sabotage you. Meal planning and food preparation are key. Drink water regularly and often. The best outcome for me was that losing the weight increased our energy, improved our health, changed our appearance and changed our way of thinking about food. I couldn't ask for anything more.

Lanna Forrest
50-year-old African-American female

Most of my life I had never been "too fat," so I was surprised when I started to seriously gain weight in 2002. Looking back, I can see that a number of things contributed to my condition. I changed jobs and was now sitting in one spot for hours. Also, I had to drive to the new job and park in a garage just outside the building. Previously, I parked a relatively long distance from the pick-up stop and had to walk six blocks to get to work. My husband became too ill to work, and my child started kindergarten and had a hard time adjusting to a class. My favorite pet, which I had walked faithfully every day, regardless of the weather, passed away. My mom was also aging, and on top of all of these concerns, I myself was aging, and losing weight was becoming harder to do.

The weight just kept adding up. Every week at the checkout counter in the grocery store, I would pick up the latest exercise/women/ladies magazine with the "greatest diet" advertised on the front. I would work at the diet faithfully for a week or two, but with no good results. Some of the articles suggested that medication may have been the culprit, and by this time I was taking three heavy duty blood pressure-lowering medications. Some of my medications did have an impact on metabolism, so I had my physician change them. The result was not very encouraging. I was a little less tired, but still sitting at an impossible weight.

Then, in May 2009, I noticed that a good friend of mine seemed to be melting away. For a number of months, she would only tell me that she was eating less. When I returned from vacation (in Hawaii, where I had to wear a mumu), she finally told me that she was seeing a doctor in Burke: Dr. Posner. By then, she had shrunk to a really swanky size. So I had what I needed to at least try the program: living proof that the program worked for someone.

I started the program on a Wednesday in August 2009. I remember thinking that I really liked the combination of foods on the plan. It was mid-summer and I had a decent-sized garden that was producing most of the vegetables listed. I was not a bread or pasta fan, so not eating these items during the induction phase of the diet was not a big deal for me. The diet supplements and medications were great too. The serotonin seemed to quell my appetite and the phentermine gave me a great boost, without too much jitteriness.

I did have some bumps in the road, especially the first weekend. I missed snacking and the taste of snacks. We kept bags of chips at home (potato chips, corn chips, Doritos), as well as at least 4 gallons of ice cream in the refrigerator. Over the years, I had developed a bad habit of snacking when I worked, so every time I sat down at the computer, my hands were accustomed to going for a chip. I had also snacked every night with my husband just before going to bed. He would offer me a "small bowl" every night. So my first weekend on the diet was hard. I must have consumed at least a pound or two of carrots for my snacks! I was not hungry, but my body literally felt like it was crying, and only the right snack would do. I had to talk to myself like a child. I reminded myself of how good my friend was looking. I pulled out the pictures from Hawaii and flipped through them. I noticed that there were not a lot of pictures of me (camera avoidance), but the ones that were there showed a very big person. I also found I could get by the cravings by leaving my office and going to bed. So I really caught up on my sleep over the next few days.

And then I met Dr. Posner at my first weigh-in. He was so encouraging. And to my great amazement, I, for whom nothing had worked for ages, had lost weight. I believe I lost between 4 and 5 pounds that first week, and I was *ecstatic*. Over the next 11 weeks, I continued to drop a pound or more every week. By the end of the 12 weeks, I had lost around 30 pounds, and I decided to sign up for an additional 6 weeks. I also have to say that the staff working the front office was great! They greeted me by name, smiled when I came in and offered to help me anyway that they could. I never left without an appointment for the next week and the paperwork I needed to file with my insurance. In 18 weeks, I ended up losing over 50 pounds.

This diet *worked* for me. I needed to see results sooner than later; and on this plan, I lost weight every single week. I love a challenge and the weekly weigh-ins provided that and a level of accountability. As I lost weight, I gained more energy and I started to feel much better about myself. One of the best things of all is the shopping that I have had to do almost every 3 weeks. One week I was wearing a size 22/24 and I was pinning them so they would not fall to the floor. When I tried on several new outfits, I was shocked to find that I wore a size 18. I had lost 6 dress sizes, and the joy of leaving the 20s behind is hard to describe. Even more amazing, I had been wearing the size 18 for only a week when I had to put a pin in the waist to keep it up! I retired those 18s at least 2 weeks ago and purchased clothes in my current size of 14/16. I am still a large, but there are no X's in front of the L!

Every female on my staff has been dieting lately. There was never so much lettuce and carrots on the fifth floor of our building. Even my friend who started on the diet earlier and introduced me to the plan has perked up her efforts, as I get closer to her size. Additionally, I have received so many compliments. My HR business partner was helping me to staff some open positions. The third time he came by my office, he stopped and apologized and said that he didn't even recognize me anymore! My family had the same reaction this past week when I went home.

Some advice I have for others is that if you have exhausted all of your food allotment for the day, find a way to hold out. Eat some of the "free items" like pickles, tomatoes, or lettuce. Try to wait a few minutes to see if you are really hungry. Try drinking something. Many times, I was really thirsty, when I thought I was hungry. Break the mold that is associated with whatever you want to eat. I went to bed early so I could get away from my desk and computer. Weigh everything that you eat. Keep a food diary, which may be hard at moments. But I look back over my diary, and I can clearly see that I am not starving myself (which is what my body/mind was saying).

Put up a picture of the new you. I have severe camera avoidance. So when I was contacted recently to provide information about my group for an article in our company's magazine, I wanted to refuse, but could not. After the interview and the picture shoot, I asked if I could have copies of the pictures. I knew I had to see them myself before they were placed where my 140,000 fellow workers would see them. I was shocked out of my wits when I saw them. I had become one of the smallest people in my group! I now use those pictures as a screen saver at work.

Kaely Clapper
16-year-old Caucasian female

My mom has struggled with weight all of her life, and she did not want me to go through the same thing. Losing weight was a "mom and daughter" endeavor that we did together, since both of us needed to lose weight. It was almost like a competition for us, but a healthy one! This was not my first attempt at losing weight. I had lost 10 pounds by myself in 3 months, but it was very hard. Staying away from the food I loved was the hardest part. So, the serotonin supplement I had as part of the Serotonin-Plus Weight Loss Program helped greatly in that sense. I wasn't feeling the same hunger for carbohydrates, which was the problem when I tried to do the Atkins diet. Although the Atkins diet helped me with weight loss, it was a very slow process. On *this* dietary plan, I never felt hungry.

The most difficult hurdles for me to overcome were self-acceptance and just being happy with myself. I knew that I needed to lose the weight for myself, because it was something I wanted to do. I have a very thin sister and have always struggled to lose weight to be more like her. Throughout my journey, my mom was a great source of support, as were the compliments from others. My friends would say, "Oh my gosh, what are you doing? You look great!" Hearing those kinds of comments really gave me the motivation to continue a healthier lifestyle.

I ended up losing 28.2 pounds in 12 weeks, and have kept it off for more than 2 months. The clinical staff was very supportive in helping me achieve my goal, and they never said anything demeaning if I had a bad week. They always had a smile to welcome me! It was helpful to have weekly weigh-ins because the weight number was presented to you formally. If I hit a plateau it just made me work harder. Before this program, I would exercise only 2 days a week. Having my mom as a workout buddy helped a lot in the beginning to get me to exercise more. I would exercise with my mom, and she would ask if I was ready to go, but I always had one more thing to do. Now I work out 6 times a week but I don't need a buddy for motivation.

I feel more alive than ever before. I just feel amazing and full of energy. I am never tired during the day and my attitude has improved toward everything. The hardest part was getting started the first week, especially giving up my usual high-carbohydrate snack foods as well as greasy, fried foods. Now I look at those foods and think, how could I ever have eaten that? I now never drink soda or eat rolls or breads. If I want a sandwich, I choose a wrap instead.

The best advice I can give is to tell people that it's not going to be a quick fix because it's a whole lifestyle change, which takes time, but the end result is amazing. You won't envy other people anymore, you will envy yourself! You will like what you see in the mirror and feel better. It is all about implementing a healthy lifestyle change that will let you feel great for years to come and be happy for the years to come, knowing you will not have to struggle with weight as you age and that you will live longer! The best part of doing this program was the lifestyle change. I went from feeling depressed to a confident, happy person!

Doug Wooddell
50-year-old Caucasian male

I have been up and down the weight chart for several years now. I cannot remember if I have ever been called or considered slim, even when I was very young. I am now over 50 years old, and I realize that if I don't get healthy, and remain so, I won't have a chance to live a long, healthy life. I want to see my children grow up (they are teenagers now), and I want to be able to see my grandchildren and be healthy enough to enjoy them.

Over the years, I have lost and regained weight several times. You name the program, and I bet I've tried it: Weight Watchers, Atkins, South Beach and Nutrisystem. They all worked to a degree, but I have always returned to being overweight.

The most difficult thing about weight loss, in general, is how much food is integrated into our society. Food is served at all gatherings and meetings, and if you are a guest at one of these, you cannot control what type of food is being served. I overcame this problem by trying to plan ahead and have good choices available to me. My family was helpful by providing healthy alternatives during the holidays. The full support from my family and friends made my endeavor much easier. I lost 54 pounds between July 22 and November 11, 2009.

The positive counseling sessions from Dr. Posner and his staff every week were enormously helpful, and stopping in the office on a weekly basis helped keep me accountable for my actions, good or bad. Knowing that in a couple of days I would be officially weighed helped me to make good decisions on several occasions. The high-protein, low-fat, lower-carbohydrate nutrition plan was sustainable and satisfying. I would say that the high-protein diet is a safe, sane diet and is relatively easy for me to stay on. I definitely felt more energy as I lost weight and continued my workout regimen.

I can't say enough how much exercise helped; it is key. Bicycling, walking, treadmill and weightlifting are some of my regular activities. Dealing with the occasional cravings was the hardest part but it was all worth it. I had hypertension and was on medications to treat it. I also was on Lipitor to reduce my cholesterol. Because of the weight loss and my new workout regimen, I now have normal blood pressure and my cholesterol went down by almost 100 points. I am now completely off the blood pressure and cholesterol-lowering medications. Overall, the weight loss itself and the way I feel are great. And I love the compliments!

Vivian Turnelle
40-year-old Caucasian female

I made the choice to lose weight because I wanted to be healthy again. My old photos from the days when I was an aerobics instructor inspired me to start a healthier lifestyle. I had been an instructor for 5 years and I loved it. Diabetes and cancer runs in my family, so it was time to get healthy for preventative health reasons. My sister had cancer, and I needed to do this for my own health and prevent the same thing from happening to me.

This was not my first attempt at losing weight. I had tried Weight Watchers in the past, but the point system did not work easily for me. I would often underestimate how many points I was eating and I didn't go to the weekly check-ins. I felt like they didn't care if I went or not. I lost a few pounds on Jenny Craig but I got bored with their prepackaged foods and it did not seem sustainable. If I veered from their foods, even a little bit, my weight loss would stall. It was very limiting and did not seem reasonable that I could only eat their foods for the rest of my life.

I loved the Serotonin-Plus Weight Loss Program once I started it and I wanted to make it work. My work environment was the most difficult obstacle to overcome, not the other stuff that many people find challenging, like avoiding a specific food, managing going out with friends, eliminating alcohol or emotional eating. I overcame my difficulty by planning and preparing to have what I needed, when I needed it. I take a cooler with meals and snacks if I won't be in an office with a refrigerator. I pack snacks like low-fat beef jerky and protein bars that I can throw in my bag when I'm on the go. Finding other options that do not derail my success has kept me going strong.

The clinic staff is *always* positive and encouraging. In addition, I had support from my family, friends, and especially my husband, who were all so motivating. My husband had lost 135 pounds on his own through a healthy lifestyle change and always encouraged me to do the same. I've known him since I was 10, so he has seen me thin and now at my heaviest.

A few helpful things the program included were the lists of foods to choose from, the exchange system and learning how to count grams of protein in terms of exchanges when looking at food labels. The advanced scale that shows weight, muscle, fat, water, body mass index, percent body fat and basal metabolic rate is informative, and it's encouraging to see these numbers improve. The serotonin and phentermine truly gave me a motivational jump-start to losing weight. I was depressed due to my sister's death from cancer, and the medications gave me the will-power to believe in it and keep going. Having a positive attitude is one of the discoveries I have made that makes a huge difference. I try not to get overwhelmed by the large amount of weight I have to lose (150 pounds), but take it gradually by reaching mini-goals; every 10 pounds has been important. Take it day by day and exercise! I lose a lot more weight when I include exercise. It really is key and goes hand-in-hand with eating healthy for weight loss. I feel better I guess because of the endorphin rush. It also helps me decompress from the day. Remember to eat all of your snacks to prevent from getting too hungry, and be sure to make them healthy choices!

At the beginning, I was worried about reducing my carbo-hydrate intake, but the serotonin and phentermine really helped decrease my appetite for these foods. I'm never hungry as long as I'm eating the way I should, the way my body wants me to. As long as I stay on schedule and stick to the program, I feel great. I have a ton more energy now from losing weight! I can go up the stairs faster now than I used to, I can actually walk *with* my husband and he doesn't have to wait for me. It's the best feeling in the world!

My most helpful tips for others on the program are that you need to give it a chance and stick with it because it really does work. I have dealt with my weight problem for over 10 years and tried everything. Slowly but surely, you will feel better in your health, your life, and attitude. You don't feel hungry on this program. I feel better about myself. I get compliments all the time from people I haven't seen in a while. They tell me I look so good and say things like, "Wow, you look awesome," which is a *great* feeling.

14. Weight Control and Mood

By Robert B. Posner, M.D.

It is safe to say that almost everyone can relate to the issue of "emotional eating". For many people, when they are happy and feeling exhilaration, food and/or alcohol are ingested in robust amounts. Conversely, for others, feelings of darkness and despair will lead to eating/gorging on high caloric food/drink sources in an attempt to elevated the depressed mood. Why do mood changes, either high or low, lead to derailing eating behaviors? Why is the hunger sensation not the only feeling that governs our eating behaviors?

Let's first break this down to gender issues: Are females more prone to "stress eating" than males? A study from Finland followed 5000 men and women and the conclusion of the study was that women are significantly are more apt than men to turn to food as a "self-treatment" for mood issues. Men are more likely to smoke cigarettes or drink alcohol as a response to depression and/or anxiety. My experience treating patients at the Serotonin-Plus weight control program is very consistent with this study result. I have found that an overwhelming majority of females report "stress/emotional" eating as a major causative factor of their weight issues. Men much more frequently tell me that the major cause is a slowing down of their metabolism as they have gotten older.

So the question becomes why do females experience stress/emotional eating much more so than males? I believe the answer is found in the neurochemical (brain chemicals) differences between the sexes as well as some environmental, social, societal and genetic contributions. Let's first focus on some of the chemicals involved.

One of the major biochemical reactions to stress is the release of a number of chemicals and hormones. If you have ever been in an accident or near accident, you may have experienced a pounding heartbeat, sweats, tremors and feeling very alert. These occur because of the release of the "flight or right" chemicals such as epinephrine (adrenaline), norepinephrine, cortisol and to some extent, insulin. Going back to our ancestral genetic roots, this "flight or fight" response was protective to an extent. When being charged by a wild animal or hostile intruder, being more alert, having the heart pick up pace and garnering strength rapidly would increase the chances of survival.

In the modern era, the stress usually does not take the form of a wild animal about to rip into your flesh or some guy with a spear targeting the central part of your chest. More often, the stress occurs because your boss is burying you with work, you child has to be at soccer practice at 5 PM, the traffic on the Beltway is horrendous and your mother in law is about to visit for 2 weeks. This modern day stress is more of a chronic situation as opposed to an acute, life or death stress. This chronic stress is more apt to cause chronic chemical changes as opposed to the acute, life-threatening stress situations that result in an immediate "burst" of these chemicals that quickly recedes when the stress situation resolves.

Cortisol, also known as "the stress hormone" is involved in a number of reactions that affect weight and body fat distribution. Cortisol is a steroid hormone produced in the adrenal glands. The functions of cortisol include:

- Elevating blood sugar (glucose) levels

- Fat, protein and carbohydrate metabolism to maintain blood glucose (gluconeogenesis)
- Immune responses
- Anti-inflammatory actions
- Blood pressure
- Heart and blood vessel tone
- Central nervous system activation

Cortisol production is influenced by the pituitary gland in the brain. The pituitary releases a number of hormones that effect peripheral glands and organs such as the thyroid, ovaries, kidneys, testes and adrenal gland. Disorders of the pituitary and/or the adrenal gland may lead to altered cortisol release.

Focusing on cortisol effects on weight control and body fat distribution, examples of these can be seen in situations when the body either markedly overproduces cortisol (an example is Cushing's Disease) and when corticosteroids are prescribed for health conditions such as refractory asthma, certain chronic skin diseases and autoimmune diseases such as Systemic Lupus Erythematosis ("Lupus") or Crohn's Disease/Ulcerative Colitis (Inflammatory bowel). The affected person will develop "moon facies" (a rounding of the facial appearance), a "buffalo hump" (fat deposited on the back below the neck), weight gain (especially around the core body) and poor blood sugar control. Clearly cortisol has effects on weight control but the question is whether chronic stress produces chronic cortisol overproduction leading to weight gain?

A study of 100 people in 1998 demonstrated that chronic stress did, in fact, lead to more chronic elevations of morning cortisol levels and this was more pronounced in females as opposed to males. However this study did not look specifically at weight control in chronically stressed people. Searching the plethora of papers written about the stress-cortisol-weight gain connection, it is not at all apparent that weight gain, can in fact, be attributed to cortisol effects produced by chronic stress. There have been many products sold in the over the counter market that purportedly produce "weight loss" by reducing cortisol but the FTC has pretty much shut down these companies because of false claims.

So, if stress-induced cortisol overproduction is not the explanation for stress eating/weight gain, what other explanation(s) are possible? Here is one from "Dr. Posner": After seeing patients for well over 30 years, I have found that almost like a reflex, the human body/mind attempts to obtain something positive when confronted with something negative. The infant gets hungry, starts crying, the mother immediately feeds the baby and satiation/quiet occurs. The adult comes home stressed from work and the "immediate gratification" will occur in the form of "few glasses of wine" and/or some high caloric food sources.

Another biochemical explanation to stress eating can be attributed to neurotransmitter imbalances. As this book is about serotonin, let's start with this brain chemical. Low serotonin levels lead to mood disorders such as depression and anxiety. Additionally, carbohydrate cravings are linked to serotonin imbalance. Chronic stress has been shown to deplete serotonin levels. The brain produces serotonin from tryptophan, an amino acid found in large amounts in dark chocolates and other high-caloric foods. Yes, tryptophan is found in proteins but the cravings for carbohydrates have some basis on the brain seeking ways to manufacture more serotonin. When serotonin levels are lowered due to stress, which in turn, can lead to depression and anxiety. This will often lead to the "immediate gratification" behavior patterns (here comes the wine and chocolates!) that will derail weight control efforts.

There is also a "chicken or the egg" issue involved with mood issues and weight control problems. If the first issue is the weight control as opposed to stress/depression/anxiety, perhaps the weight control problem is *causing* the stress/mood issues as opposed to the weight gain being *caused by* the stress/mood issues. Overweight /obese people tend to have a multitude of medical and psychological ramifications such as:

- Metabolic problems such as diabetes mellitus
- Organ-specific issues such as heart disease
- Chronic pain syndromes
- Sleep apnea
- Gastrointestinal problems
- Low self-esteem
- Low self-confidence
- Social withdrawal

These physical and emotional conditions will cause almost anyone to feel stressed. With more stress comes more cortisol production, more serotonin depletion, etc. This "vicious cycle" will result in ever-increasing numbers on the scale until either of the initiating conditions is resolved. We have seen over and over in the Serotonin-Plus Program that when weight control occurs, peoples' moods are improved exponentially. It is often amazing to see how quickly aggressive weight control results in a mood "makeover". I have seen many, many cases of people that break down crying during their first visits because of the emotional turmoil/sadness that the weight situation has caused and within one week, the entire demeanor changes. Often, by the end of the doctor office visit phase of the program, patients leave with some of the biggest smiles I have ever seen.

What is the best approach to addressing mood issues affecting weight control or, conversely, weight control affecting mood issues? Here are my recommendations:

- First, try to identify if there is some "fixable" chemical imbalance causing the mood issues. Medical conditions such as thyroid imbalance, adrenal gland dysfunction, vitamin deficiencies and other organic issues could impact mood as well as weight. See your primary care physician to express your concerns and hopefully the doctor will perform and examination and laboratory blood testing that will identify the imbalance and then be enact a treatment plan to correct this.

- Perform a self-assessment analysis to see if you are experiencing depression. A commonly used self-assessment is the Zung Self Rating Depression Scale (**http://healthnet.umassmed.edu/mhealth/ZungSelfRate dDepressionScale.pdf**). If the assessment indicates a diagnosis of depression, visit your physician to discuss options for treatment.

- Join a support group and this does not mean that you need to show up to some school/church auditorium, wear a badge with your first name and have everyone there in unison say "Hi _____" There are many online resources to be able to receive support from people going through many of the same issues you are going through. These online resources provide lots of anonymity and convenience.

- Try to take a few seconds delay before the act of reaching for a food/drink source in response to a mood issue. I ask my patients to carry with them a 3X5 card bullet pointing the 4 or 5 major reasons why it is so important for them to control weight. When confronted with a stress/emotional eating situation, take that card out, read through the list and then make the decision after this delay: Is the food/drink *really* going to help the situation?

In conclusion, there is no doubt that mood issues are intricately involved in our eating/drinking behaviors and conversely, our eating/drinking behaviors can have profound effects on our moods. Recognition of this complex interplay is the first step in being able to address these issues in a way necessary to maintain a healthy weight AND a healthy emotional state. Is this easy to achieve? Of course not. Is it possible? Absolutely YES!!!

15. One Last Word

By Robert Posner, M.D. and Donna L. Eckenrode, MPAS, PA-C

The Serotonin-Plus Weight Loss program addresses the underlying chemical problems that make weight loss difficult, while providing a sustainable nutritional plan using real food. Unlike other programs, it is not a diet. Nor is it a miracle program based on a magic pill. We do provide patients with supplements, Serotonin-Plus Weight Management Formula and Serotonin-Plus Multivitamin supplements, to manage carbohydrate and sugar cravings, but they are part of a larger concept that includes exercise, careful eating and personal accountability. The title of this book is *The Serotonin Solution to Never "Dieting" Again*, not *Serotonin-Plus, the Magic Diet Pill.*

The Serotonin-Plus method encourages patients to make lifestyle modifications that allow them to reach their weight loss goals while also providing them with strategies for long-term weight management. These lifestyle modifications are maintainable, improve the quality of life and happiness and help prevent and manage weight gain.

The preceding chapters have laid out the basic nature of weight gain, weight loss and weight maintenance, and they have established some fundamental points that must always be kept in mind. Successful weight loss efforts and weight maintenance require intentionality: you must think about what you are doing. You must plan to live in a healthy way, which means not only eating properly but staying physically active. Instead of reflexively going to the local fast-food restaurant to pick up dinner after a busy day at work, or sitting on the couch with a glass of wine in the evenings, you have to keep your focus by planning ahead for the week's meals and exercise schedule. Challenge yourself daily by asking, "What am I going to do today in order to be healthy?" Always be aware of your weight by weighing in weekly, at home, and treating a gain of 5 pounds as you would a gain of 30 pounds.

Maintaining focus and energy on your weight loss or maintenance efforts is easier said than done, and even this book can take you only so far. For extra assistance, read Dr. Posner's daily blog to get a dose of encouragement and strategies for managing common pitfalls. Visit our website (www.spdiet.com) to make an appointment at one of our clinics or to purchase supplements. If you are a former patient and need assistance with management or want to restart your weight loss efforts, we would be very pleased to see you again. We are here to help you, not judge you, and we understand that it is not easy to maintain a healthy weight.

There is nothing fun about the act of losing weight. What is fun about cutting down on food and drink sources that provide us an immediate gratification? What is fun about waking yourself up 30 minutes earlier 4 times a week to exercise before work? What is fun about being around a bunch of friends at a restaurant that are pouring the wine and ordering desserts and you are shaking your head saying "no thanks"? What is *fun* is looking younger, living longer, having more energy, fitting into those beautiful clothes that have been gathering dust in the closet, ridding yourself of medications for diabetes, high blood pressure and elevated cholesterol levels, having less back and joint pain, not needing a sleep apnea mask, enjoying quality time with your loved ones and having infinite more confidence and self-esteem. These are what successful weight control brings you. Compare those to the immediate gratifica-

tion of inanimate food/drink sources and your choice becomes quite clear: Lose the weight and keep it off.

Selections from Dr. Posner's Blog

By Robert B. Posner, M.D.

Every morning I wake up and one of my first actions is to write my daily blog entry. I started this about 5 years ago and I continue to do this. Our patients often laugh at the typographical errors, slang and some of the other aspects of these daily musings that should not be confused with great medical writing.

At last count, there are well over 1600 entries I have written and although I cannot claim the Cal Ripken-ish, never missing a day "record streak", I pretty much do this 7 days a week, 52 weeks a year. I dare say that there is no other doctor that communicates daily with his/her patients in this manner.

The reason why I do this every day: As a practicing physician for over 30 years, and having seen and continue to see many thousands of patients for weight control, I have learned that people need a tremendous amount of support in their weight loss journey from start to NEVER finishing. Now, that last sentence was not good English, but I wanted to drive home the point that there is no "finish line" to a long- term weight control journey. Yes, there may be a "start" date, but we cannot target a completion date, as to do so will result in the classic "yo-yo dieting".

People need support along the way, not only during the active weight losing phase, but even more importantly, when goals have been reached maintenance is required. When patients are coming to the Serotonin-Plus Weight Loss Program, everyone loses lots of weight. The reasons? 1- We are providing appetite suppressants 2- We see patients once a week 3- People are paying lots of money to join our program. When people complete their formal programs, what is left as far as support? The answer is that I view my blog as a supportive tool that hopefully serves as a daily reminder/inspiration to help the person make choices that day that will be better suited for weight control. I would love to have my patients hear my voice echo in the mind every day reminding them of the importance of their successful weight control efforts.

There are so many events, situations, people, issues etc. that divert attention from taking care of ourselves. To lose weight and keep that weight off, we MUST be able to spend time planning meals, carving out exercise time, shopping at the right places and otherwise taking "control". As soon as we stop thinking about all the aspects of a successful weight control journey, I guarantee you that all of the weight will return. As I tell my patients, if you were making a bet in Las Vegas about a chronically overweight/obese person losing the weight AND keeping the weight off, take the side of the bet that has the person failing. However, I want ALL of my patients to be "Winners" in the battle, hence my daily message as a potential supportive tool.

As I plan to keep writing these entries every day, please feel free to send us your e-mail address and we can send this message daily to you or just log on to **www.spdiet.com** and you can find the blog tab on the home page. I also really like when people send me comments on the subject matter I write about, debate me on my opinions etc. Happy reading!

Being in the Weight Loss "Zone"

Every week patients come back to our program who have been with us previously. Each one of them did very well in their first program with us, losing weight aggressively and leaving quite happy. However, over a period of months or years, for a significant number of people, weight will start going up again. In a perfect world, our program or anyone else's for that matter would help people lose weight permanently.

Unfortunately, lifestyle changes that relate to food consumption, alcohol usage and exercise (or lack thereof) are very difficult to accomplish permanently. Temporarily, we can go on "diets," meaning for a *period of time* we change our behavioral patterns, but a very common psychological factor is our desire to cross a finish line. When we have reached our goal or close to it, we start going back to old behaviors.

Truly, to lose weight and keep it off requires lifestyle changes and permanent behavior modification. When people decide to start a weight loss effort, they are in a mental zone of sorts, meaning they are geared up mentally to alter their lifestyle.

Weight Loss and "the Last Straw"

For many, it will take a "last straw" to become motivated and begin a healthier lifestyle. Yesterday I had two patients who described their reason for entering our program. For one, it was being placed by her internist on a blood pressure medication. The other said that she put on one of her favorite dresses and it did not fit. In one case, it was a health issue that caused the patient to make a definitive move. In the other, it was an aesthetic/vanity motivator.

When it comes to confronting a weight problem, many people take the road of denial/avoidance. They do not check their weight, avoid looking in the mirror and in general block out thoughts of addressing the weight problem. However, when something very real happens, such as a medical problem requiring medication or other intervention, or a social situation calls for the wearing of a gown or a bathing suit, they are forced to confront their weight issue.

For some, the last straw may come too late: a serious heart attack or a major diabetic complication. *Now* is the time to do something about your weight. Do not wait for a last straw!

War versus Battle

When patients come in for their weekly visits and some weight gain has occurred, we ask them to understand that not every week will be successful. Due to factors like business travel or personal stress, sometimes focus is lost a bit, and when that happens, a weight gain will occur. Remember that a weight gain for a week does not make you a failure. Gather your forces and focus, and make the next week more aggressive. The war is an assault on the excessive weight that puts you at health risk and also makes you not feel good about yourself. Each day is a battle, and some days the battle will not go completely in your favor. That's okay. The big picture is the long-term reduction of the weight and all the positive effects that it brings.

Keep fresh in your mind the reasons why you committed yourself to losing weight. Our instinctual behavior patterns will often make these reasons blur a bit, but if you can marshal your forces to keep the reasons clear and at the forefront of your mind, it will be easier to say no to the food that will harm you.

Remember the Reasons Why....

I saw one patient yesterday who started the program at a very obese weight and within 15 weeks lost almost 80 pounds. He was telling me that he recently returned from a family vacation and was able to play with his children in the ocean, something he had not been able to do previously because of his weight. As he was interacting with his family, he started thinking that his efforts will allow him to spend many more years providing resources for his family as well as being able to spend time with them. He began to feel an obligation to his children and wife to lose the weight. He felt that it was selfish on his part to have allowed himself to reach a medically dangerous weight.

I saw another patient yesterday who has lost over 30 pounds, with her major motivation being her daughter's wedding. Originally it was all about looking great in her dress. However, over the last month or so, she started realizing that she had been suffering from a global lack of self-esteem, and that the significant weight loss had increased her confidence and positive feelings about herself.

The bottom line: there is nothing "fun" about losing weight. It means giving up or altering behavior patterns that are pleasurable and hedonistic. But the results are being healthier, living longer, avoiding debilitating diseases, looking younger, having higher levels of self-confidence and rediscovering your ego. These *are* fun. Focus on the reasons why you want to lose weight and keep them at the forefront of your mind. This may allow you to "just say no" to the treats and goodies which are the saboteurs and hurtful things to our health.

Staying Healthy

As you enjoy the company of your friends, family and loved ones, give special thanks, if you have relatively good health, for the fact that you are there in a pretty good state to enjoy your family time. In my internal medicine practice, I see many cases of people who have the sudden onset of significant medical problems that have a good chance of shortening their lifespan. They will enjoy fewer Christmas dinners with their families. It is sad.

What shortens a person's lifespan? Heart disease, diabetes, cancers. What contributes to the development of heart disease, diabetes, breast cancer, pancreatic cancer and colon cancer? Obesity.

Losing weight is certainly going to help you aesthetically, but for living life to the fullest and being there to see your children and grandchildren grow and flourish, there is nothing better you can do for yourself. Life often is a series of choices. Choosing to be there with your loved ones, versus eating high-calorie food or alcohol, is a better choice.

Serotonin Science

Weight Control and Brain Chemicals

The book I wrote a book several years ago was about serotonin and how its imbalance can affect a number of body systems.

It is amazing how the slightest imbalance of a chemical that is present in such small amounts can have such life-altering effects. The total body content of serotonin is about 10 mg (the size of a small Claritin tablet), and most of it is found in the gastrointestinal tract. In the brain, concentrations of serotonin are minute, yet the subtlest imbalances may lead to severe depression, anxiety and other significant mood disorders.

We inherit brain chemical imbalances. As with mood disorders, we often inherit weight-control and metabolism issues, cravings and other factors that result in excess weight. When obesity runs rampant in our family, we ask whether this is environmental versus genetic. Some families, more than others, base their family gatherings and shows of nurture by providing more high-calorie foods. This is the environmental component. Slow metabolism or a tendency toward addictive behaviors is more the chemical contributor. Both play a large role in familial obesity.

The solutions involve changing the customary routine of feeding family members beyond reason, and consciously counting calories/portions or in some other way limiting caloric intake. Certainly, a program such as ours can help focus people on these issues. That is why I constantly tell patients that pills are only an adjunct to a long-term strategy for weight loss. Changing behaviors and finding adaptive ways to mitigate negative brain chemical contributions to eating patterns are the necessary components for long-term weight loss.

Serotonin Depletion and Cravings

Part of the stress-eating issue and the explanation as to why we crave sweets, chocolates and carbohydrates when we are stressed can be explained by serotonin depletion.

Okay, now to the boring biochemistry lesson and explanation. The brain produces serotonin from the amino acid *tryptophan*. Amino acids are the basic building block of proteins and are present in our diet. Tryptophan is found in turkey and chicken, but large amounts are present in sweets and carbohydrates. During times of serotonin depletion, such as periods of high stress or a woman's menstrual cycle, the brain needs to manufacture more serotonin. Signals are then sent out that make us seek the foods that have the building block, tryptophan. Unfortunately, the food sources that contain the tryptophan are the high-caloric sweets and carbohydrates. Hence, the reasoning for the development and use of the Serotonin-Plus supplement that increases serotonin levels, therein decreasing cravings for carbohydrates.

What Are Empty Calories?

With barbecues, vacations and beach trips around every corner of your summer, you may have read the term empty calories or heard it used by nutritionists or even TV talk-show hosts. But what exactly are empty calories? Why are they so bad for you, and how can you avoid them?

Empty calories = high calories but low nutrition. Empty calories are also known as "junk food" because they lack health-promoting nutrients.

Examples of foods containing mostly empty calories:

French fries, fried chicken, chips and all other deep-fried foods. A large order of fries from a fast-food chain can contain up to 570 calories with 30g of *total fat* and 8g of *trans-fat*.

Candy, soda and other sweetened packaged foods. A can of soda contains about 130 calories as well as additives and colorings.

Beer, wine and all other alcoholic beverages. A can of beer contains about 150 calories from carbohydrates and not much of anything else. In addition, calories from alcohol tend to be stored as fat in the abdomen = beer belly.

Refined grains such as crackers, cookies, white rice and white bread. Refined grains do provide some *B vitamins*, but that's it.

How to avoid empty calories?

Avoid deep-fried foods. Instead of frying, try baking or broiling foods.

Avoid high-calorie/sugar drinks. Instead try Crystal Light flavored water or diet juices and teas.

Try whole grains instead of refined grains (white bread).

Snack on fruits or vegetables instead of potato chips.

Beware Hidden Sugars!

We all know the less sugar we consume, the better our diet is and the fewer calories we take in. Although many of us try to use low-calorie sweeteners like Splenda, Equal or Sweet N' Low, as a nation we rely on sugar. Today, the average American consumes 156 pounds of sugar per year, according to the U.S. Department of Agriculture (USDA). However, only about 29 pounds of it comes as traditional sugar, or sucrose, according to the Sugar Association, a trade group of sugar manufacturers. The rest comes from the foods we consume daily, but they are hidden. Of course, those foods include things like candy, soda and other junk foods. But plenty of sugar is hiding in places where you might not expect it. Some types of crackers, yogurt, ketchup and peanut butter, for instance, are loaded with sugar and carbohydrates. This sugar hides in the form of high-fructose corn syrup, or HFCS.

In the U.S. diet, the major source of "added sugar," not including naturally occurring sugars like the fructose in fruit, is soft drinks. According to the USDA, sweetened fruit drinks account for 10% of the total added sugars we consume. Candy and cake come in at 5% each. Ready-to-eat cereal comprises 4% of the total. The biggest chunk, making up 26% of added sugars, comes from prepared foods like ketchup, canned vegetables and fruits and peanut butter.

Another high-sugar trap can be low-fat products, which may not be as good for your diet as you think. Some contain plenty of sugar to make up for the lack of tasty fat. For instance, reduced fat peanut butter has less fat than the regular, but what you may not know is that this reduced fat brand actually has more sugar and more carbohydrates. Food marketers find ways to trick the consumer to think some products are healthier than others, by using health-conscious terms. In this case, the regular peanut butter would be the better choice, because it has the same number of calories as the reduced fat brand but lower amounts of sugar and carbohydrates. This shows that when fat is removed, it may be replaced with much higher levels of sugar and carbohydrates.

According to the USDA, between 1987 and 1997, consumption of added sugar in the United States grew 20%. This trend is also being seen in the developing world, according to the World Health Organization (WHO). That's one reason both the United Nations and the WHO released guidelines in 2003 that say sugar should account for no more than 10% of daily calories. In a daily 2,000-calorie diet, that's just 200 calories. So be mindful of the calories and total carbohydrates of your food choices. Read the nutritional labels and compare regular versus low-fat versions of products.

To keep you on track here is a list of ingredients that are considered added sugars and can increase the total carbohydrate content:

Beet sugar
Brown sugar
Cane sugar
Confectioner's sugar
Crystallized cane juice
Dextrose
Evaporated cane juice
Fructose
High-fructose corn syrup
Honey
Invert sugar
Maltodextrin (or dextrin)
Maple syrup
Molasses
Raw sugar

Sucrose (table sugar or white sugar)
Turbinado sugar

Modifying Behavior

Responding to Hunger Signals

When we recall being children or raising our small ones, we often conjure up images of children being cajoled or coerced to eat. Sometimes we were threatened with not getting dessert unless we ate our main course, or could not leave the table to play with our friends until we ate our spinach. We were usually skinny little ones with not one ounce of fat on our bodies, and if we weren't hungry, we could care less about eating "real" food. Sure, we loved candy, cakes and ice cream, but who cared about a juicy steak and potatoes?

Trying to re-learn the concept of eating in response to actual hunger is important in helping long-term weight loss. At what point does it switch over and we start making our eating choices based on issues other than hunger? At a restaurant after that appetizer, basket of warm bread, large main course and side dishes, who actually feels the concept of "hunger" when the waiter brings out that tempting dessert tray? Of course we feel no hunger, but we order a dessert anyway. Sometimes we find ourselves eating because it is "eating time," or finishing a large portion at a restaurant because we are not going directly home, the food will spoil in the car and we don't want to "waste" food.

Try this as a test. Every time you are ready to put in a mouthful of food, ask, "Am I Hungry?"

Understanding Portion Control

Most people consume far more calories than they realize. Why? They don't rationally estimate portion size. According to a survey conducted by the American Institute for Cancer Research (AICR), most Americans (78 percent) still believe that the kind of food they eat is more important in managing their weight than the amount of food they eat.

Americans are concentrating too much on cutting fat, or relying on fad diets that cut intake but lower the metabolism. Studies reveal that these strategies fail to address the issue of total calories consumed, as well as overall good nutrition. Experts say that understanding the concept of standard serving sizes is essential to good nutrition and weight maintenance. Standardized serving sizes help consumers, health professionals and food manufacturers find a common language.

Although serving sizes are standardized, individual portion sizes will vary, because people have different caloric requirements. Portion size also depends on a person's specific weight-management goals and health needs.

The problems of obesity and lack of nutrition awareness also seem to have societal and cultural components. Take a look at fast-food restaurants. Most offer "super-size" or "value" meals, which may contain an entire day's worth of calories and fat. In addition, full-service restaurants offer large portions to provide value to customers in a competitive environment. Similarly, with today's hectic pace and more women in the workforce, it is easier for many to grab ready-made or easily prepared foods like pasta that contain more carbohydrates. Statistics from the U.S. Department of Agriculture reveal that Americans' total daily caloric intake has risen by 148 calories per day since 1980. This adds an extra 15 pounds to weight every year.

Interestingly, the same studies show that the amount of fat in the average American diet has decreased from 40% of total calories to 33% during the same period. So although calories from fat have decreased, at 9 calories per gram of fat versus only 4 for a gram of carbohydrate or protein, Americans have more than made up for their lower fat intakes with larger portion sizes of other types of foods. Larger portion sizes equal more calories. And more calories lead to weight gain, regardless of the source of the calories: fat, protein or carbohydrate.

Fat provides a feeling of fullness, which can help some people avoid eating to excess. By cutting fat out of their diets, people may lose this signal to stop eating. In addition, many low-fat and no-fat foods can be just as high in calories as the regular versions because fat is replaced with sugars or high-calorie sweeteners to beef up flavor.

What constitutes a proper portion size? According to the American Dietetic Association, you can use the following "models" to approximate portion sizes:

- One deck of playing cards equals 1 serving (3 ounces) of meat, poultry or fish. (You can also use the palm of a woman's hand or a computer mouse.)

- Half a baseball equals 1 serving (½ cup) of fruit, vegetables, pasta or rice. (You can also use a small fist.)

- Your thumb equals 1 serving (1 ounce) of cheese.

- A small hand holding a tennis ball equals 1 serving (1 cup) of yogurt or chopped fresh greens.

Dining Out: To Cheat or Not to Cheat?

Dining out can be a challenge for anyone, whether we are watching our weight or not. There are so many choices. Americans dine out more than ever, and portions are larger than ever. Restaurants, however, are more accommodating to health and diet needs than they were in the past.

Think carefully about the food you are going to choose and ask yourself if the calories and setback are worth it. Here are some tips that might help you in making choices when you do eat out.

If you are busy and eat out often, avoid considering dining out a special occasion. When we think of dining out as a special occasion or celebration, we tend to overeat or indulge in foods that we might not otherwise eat.

Budget your calories throughout the day. If you know you are going out to eat for dinner, try to reduce your intake at breakfast and lunch so you can save some of your calories for when you dine out. However, you may want to have a small snack to help curb your appetite before dining out to help you avoid eating too much at your meal.

If you know where you will dine out, look up the menu (and nutrition information, if available) online and decide what you will eat before you get to the restaurant. This way you are in control to choose a lower-calorie, lower-fat meal and are not overwhelmed by the menu and careless about eating healthy when you arrive hungry at the restaurant.

Share your meal with a friend or family member. Most restaurants serve portions that are two to three times what we need. Otherwise, have the serving staff put half of the meal in a to-go box before it is brought to the table.

Avoid all the extras, as these calories add up quickly: bread and butter on the table, sweetened drinks, appetizers, side items and desserts. Instead focus on a healthy balance of lean proteins, low-fat carbohydrates and fruits and vegetables.

Alcohol and Weight Loss

Successful weight loss is all about burning more calories than you take in. In an effort to save calories when we go on a diet, many of us choose lower-calorie alcoholic drinks, mainly because they contain fewer alcohol calories than their regular counterparts. However, drinking too much has a far more damaging effect than you can imagine, by increasing caloric intake but also by reducing the number of fat calories you burn. Alcohol can increase your appetite for up to 24 hours after you finish drinking.

Research reported in the *American Journal of Clinical Nutrition* studied the metabolic effect in adult men. Each was given two drinks of vodka and sugar-free lemonade, separated by 30 minutes. Each drink contained just under 90 calories. Fat metabolism was measured before and after consumption. For several hours after drinking the vodka, fat metabolism dropped by 73%. The way your body responds to alcohol is very similar to the way it deals with excess carbohydrate.

The combination of alcohol and a high-calorie meal is especially fattening, mainly because alcohol acts as a potent appetizer. A Canadian study showed that an aperitif increased calorie intake to a greater extent than a non-alcoholic beverage. Researchers from Denmark's Royal Veterinary and Agricultural University reported similar results. When a group of men were given a meal and allowed to eat as much as they wanted, they ate more when the meal was served with beer or wine than a soft drink.

Alcohol suppresses the number of fat calories your body burns for energy much more than meals rich in protein, carbohydrate or fat. While an occasional drink isn't going to do much damage, consistent alcohol intake will reduce overall lean muscle mass, significantly lowering metabolism.

Weight Loss/Maintenance Strategies for the Summer Season

Summer is a very busy time for many of us. We have vacations and graduation parties, barbeques and weddings, to name a few. How can we lose weight or even maintain with so many things going on? Here are some tips.

1) If you are going on vacation, pack healthy, low-calorie, portable snacks like veggies, cheese or yogurt, whether you are driving or flying, so you're less likely to be tempted by unhealthy options.

2) Exercise more often and longer to expend more calories if you know you will be taking more calories in. If you increase your exercise during this time period, you'll reduce the damage of increasing your caloric intake. The more you exercise the more you can eat without gaining weight, and exercise is a great stress reliever.

3) Eat sensibly *before* you go to parties and barbeques. You'll be less likely to be tempted by goodies if you're already full.

4) When you do eat out on vacation, order a dinner salad, pass on the bread and munchies served and split an entrée with someone.

5) When heading off to parties, volunteer to be the designated driver. Alcohol provides many empty calories that you don't need. If you must drink, try a wine spritzer or, for example, a rum and diet coke. Avoid sweet frozen drinks and the sugar of regular sodas.

6) Whenever you encounter plates of food buffet-style, snack on fresh raw vegetables and lean protein, and avoid sweets and high-calorie selections. When possible,

move away from the food table. You will be less likely to be tempted to eat more.

7) Choose water or low-calorie beverages whenever possible. Avoid the empty calories of alcohol, regular soda, punch and other fruit juices. Drink water before your meal to feel full sooner.

8) Eat slowly and, if socially acceptable, chat often. If you eat slowly and talk longer, you'll be full sooner. Try to savor every bite. It takes 20 minutes for the stomach to signal to your brain that you are full. At meals, fill up on low-calorie appetizers, if possible, like salads with low-calorie dressing, raw vegetables or soups.

9) When on vacation eat your low-calorie snacks and drink your water. Avoid skipping meals.

10) Eat dessert in moderation, having a small piece or just a bite. Pass up peanuts, chips and other everyday snacks. Spend your calories on the special treats you really want. If you do need to snack choose a few pretzels or unbuttered popcorn.

11) When attending a party or barbeque, wear a form-fitting outfit, with a belt if possible, to remind you to not over-eat.

12) Make socializing, rather than food, the focus of the event. Keep your portions in check to keep calories under control.

13) Practice saying "No, thank you." It's okay to turn down invitations or tell a pushy host you don't want seconds. Stop eating when you are no longer hungry. Bring fat-free or low-fat dishes to parties. Encourage others to do the same.

14) Arrive at mealtime for a dinner party and avoid before-dinner drinks and appetizers.

15) Attend only the parties you really want to go to. You'll save a lot of calories and time.

16) If you are tempted by the frozen margaritas, make your own low-calorie frozen drink using Crystal Light, water and crushed ice.

Hopefully these tips will help you to save calories as you enjoy your summer.

How Often to Weigh Yourself?

I have patients who get on that scale several times a day and others who will weigh themselves once a week. What is the best frequency? My answer: it depends on the person.

Weight will vary daily, and not always as a result of our caloric intake. If you have a salty meal and drink lots of fluids, your weight will go up, which has nothing to do with fat. It is water weight. Female patients can relate to the fluid retention that can occur during certain times of their cycle. Their weight may go up 4-5 pounds over several days, which has nothing to do with "real" weight gain.

Keep a clipboard next to your scale and weigh and record that number once a week. Do the measurement at approximately the same time every week. Then, depending on that number, have a plan as to what you will do about it. If you know you have liberalized your alcohol and caloric intake that week, and the scale shows the damages, revert to the Phase One diet plan for the upcoming week; one week later, recheck the scale weight. *Always* have a plan when you see the weight.

We get into trouble when we either do not monitor the weight or we have no plan. Let me give you an example of the former. I had a patient who lost 68 pounds in our program in 6 months. He did a great job. He is my medical patient as well, and 3 months after exiting the weight loss program he came in for a medical appointment. I saw immediately there was significant weight gain and I asked him how much he had gained. He sheepishly said that he had reverted to some old behaviors and gained back about 15 pounds. We went to the scale and it was actually 39.4. His mind tricked him into think- ing the weight gain was fairly moderate but in fact, he gained back all of the weight he worked so hard to lose. I convinced him to monitor the weight and get back into the zone.

Weighing yourself daily may drive you a bit crazy because sometimes you will see fluctuations that will not make sense and you will become frustrated. Hence, my recommendations for a once-weekly weigh-in.

Social Pressures

Jealous Sabotage?

We frequently see patients who tell us that their friends are trying to deflect them from their weight loss efforts. When they go out with certain friends they are always being pressured to eat food or drink alcohol that would clearly hinder weight loss efforts. "Come on, a little piece of cake can't hurt you....You aren't fun anymore!"

I do not think that sabotage is truly intentional, but it certainly can make your weight loss efforts more difficult. Your attempt to lose weight may threaten others around you who also need to lose weight but show little effort. Subconsciously, the overweight person who is not showing control feels even more of a failure by watching someone around them take a proactive stance. They admire their friend's efforts, yet may feel jealous and possibly be hoping they fail. Hey, if everyone in the group is eating cheesecake for dessert, it must be okay, right? But if one or several people take a pass on dessert, those who are eating it do not have as much fun doing so.

Be firm with your friends who try to push things of high caloric content on you. Have a taste if you must, but stop there. Tell them that you are trying to lose weight and you would love their help.

Weight Loss and Disappointment

Often, when a patient comes in after a challenging week, they seem reticent about getting on the scale, not so much because they are upset, but because they feel they are letting their doctor down. I always reassure them that we feel not one bit of disappointment for a week of weight gain. We are here to help people lose weight, not judge them, and our support does not change based on that week's results.

We are all susceptible to the feeling that our actions somehow affect the way others see us. I have had many patients who do not tell anyone they are in a medical weight loss program for fear that if they leave and put weight back on, the people around them will see them as losers.

The fear of failure in front of others often motivates us to be more aggressive. Whether it be our weight loss program or any other physician's, the success comes in part from the "accountability" of knowing you have to get on that scale in front of someone else. When that someone else is a medical profession-al, a weigh-in can be an even more traumatic event in the case of no weight loss.

Your efforts to lose weight and success in reaching your goals are only for you to judge. My staff and I are here to help you achieve the results you desire. Try to eliminate thoughts that a weight-gaining week somehow disappoints us. Similar-ly, you should regard your friends, family and loved ones as support and not a panel of Olympics judges. Look at the big picture, meaning that you do not call yourself a failure after a week of weight gain. Use a week of no weight loss or gain to motivate you to gather your determination and meet the next week more aggressively.

Support Systems

It's Easier with a Partner

A husband/wife team came into my office yesterday and they have been very successful in their weight loss efforts. I was talking with them and probing how they have been so success-ful. They replied, almost simultaneously, "Doing this together makes it much easier."

When a person embarks on an initiative to lose weight, hav-ing the support of a family member, friend, co-worker or other can be incredibly helpful. When two or more people decide together to lose weight, each becomes a support group to the other. Friendly challenges such as bets on who reaches goals quicker can make it less burdensome. Having the support of someone who is doing this alongside of you can be a great motivator. If you are considering a weight loss effort, try to find someone in your world who is willing to roll up their sleeves and get to work with you.

Weight Loss and Family Members

Yesterday I saw a teenage female in our program who has not been very successful in losing weight. Her parents pressured her to start the program and the motivation was not there to begin with. Obviously, to achieve significant weight loss there must be motivation from within.

It is a delicate situation when you have a family member or friend who needs to lose weight, and although you have their best interest in mind, it seems almost presumptuous or pushy to even suggest a weight loss program. When the affected person is your child, who does not have their own monetary resources, the control is in your hands.

Young people do not worry about heart attacks, strokes or diabetes. Their motivation to lose weight is from a vanity perspective. It is difficult to address these issues with your loved ones for fear of hurting their feelings. However, not to address the issue or offer help could be deemed as irresponsible. A fine line indeed!

Social Impact

Being a Role Model and Inspiration

As you work through your weight loss efforts, others are watching and hoping you succeed. Along the way, you may become an inspiration to others. Perhaps you have children who have weight issues, or a spouse. Maybe it is a friend or co-worker who needs to lose weight, but has not yet found the fortitude to begin.

To feel that your weight loss initiative may motivate significant persons in your life almost puts more pressure on you to be successful. But when you lose a significant amount of weight and become healthier and look younger, you will serve as an inspiration to others around you. Not only are you helping yourself, but others as well.

Weight Loss and Americans

Yesterday's front page of *USA Today* carried an article detailing the extent of how obesity is costing America billions of dollars in medical care. Americans who are 30 pounds or more above a healthy body weight cost the country $147 billion in obesity-associated medical problems in 2008, and this is double the amount from 1998. Obesity accounts for 9.1% of healthcare expenditures, up from 6.5 % in 1998.

Obesity is the biggest reason for healthcare cost increases, and most of this $147 billion is being paid by taxpayers, as over 50% of the obesity-related expenditures are taking place in the Medicare and Medicaid programs.

As the President and our elected officials are working through healthcare reform, it is imperative that the obesity epidemic be addressed and steps taken to reverse this trend. Otherwise, the entire system will collapse from lack of money to pay for the services and medications required.

Weight Loss and the Future

A study released by the United Health Foundation, based on data analysis, predicts that the obesity rate in the U.S. will be 43% by 2018 and that Americans will be spending $343 billion on obesity-related health issues by that year. The obesity rate has risen 129% in the past 20 years.

Whenever we see these types of numbers, we feel alarmed, but I am not certain if we all understand just how devastating this trend will be. If we think there is a healthcare crisis now, wait until a third of the population has diabetes with all of the co-morbidities associated with it. Rationing of healthcare? Bet on it! There is no way the generation after the baby boomers will be able to afford the taxes to support Medicare and other government healthcare programs. Healthcare expenditures will rise exponentially, and people will be going without medications. Many will not be able to see a doctor. Throw on top of this the critical shortage of primary care physicians and we are setting up a frightening situation.

The above sounds like the little kid screaming that the sky is falling. But the data is real, and this is what the future holds if we cannot, as a society, put a brake on this situation.

Sources

Most of the information in this book comes from experience gained at the Serotonin-Plus Clinics. Additionally, we consulted published scientific and other expert research for certain topics, as noted below.

Chapter 1, Introduction

The $343 billion estimate of obesity-related health problems by the year 2018 comes from Partnership to Fight Chronic Disease (2009).

Chapter 3, The Serotonin Connection

For the history of serotonin's discovery and a discussion of its importance to bodily functions, see Posner (2004).

Chapter 4, Who is to Blame for America's Most Significant Health Issue?

The statistics on the general U.S. public are drawn from Flegal et al. (2010), Centers for Disease Control (2008) and O'Callaghan (2009). For adult obesity see also American Public Health Association (November 2009).

Chapter 5, African-Americans and Weight Loss

The figures for obesity among African-Americans come from Office of Minority Health (October 21, 2009). For African-American women the data are from Ogden et al. (2007) and Office of Minority Health (2009). The socioeconomic disparity between African-Americans and Caucasian-Americans has been well documented; see Office of Minority Health (October 21, 2009). Additional useful reports include Becker et al. (November 2, 2004), Office of Minority Health (December 15, 2009) and Minority Women's Health (March 2008).

Chapter 6, Weight Loss and the Menopausal Female

On the origin of "perimenopause," see Kohrt (2009). For the role of estrogen in the production of serotonin, see McEwen (2002). The statement that women using hormone-replacement therapy gain less weight than those who do not is based on Kohrt (2009). The relationship between short-term hormone suppression and a decrease in metabolic rate is also discussed by Kohrt (2009).

Chapter 9, The Essential Guide to Eating on the Serotonin-Plus Weight Loss Program

Mahan and Escott-Stump (2008) is the main source for the discussion of fats (pp. 59, 54), carbohydrates (43, 47), whole fruits and vegetables (858), the importance of drinking water (145) and the role of alcohol in reducing metabolism (713, 59). For the omega-3 and omega-6 polyunsaturated fatty acids, see Simopoulos (2008). See also Psota et al. (2006).

Deep pigmentation as an indicator of fruits and vegetables that contain high levels of antioxidants is covered by International Food Information Council Foundation (2009). For phytochemicals, see American Heart Association (2010). The relationship among consumption of carbohydrates, glycogen depletion and fat metabolism is discussed by Westman et al. (2007). For the importance of fiber-packed complex carbohydrates, see Wilson (2008). The recommendations on daily fiber needs are presented by Martlett et al. (2008). For the Institute of Medicine recommendations on water see Institute of Medicine

(2004). The diabetic exchange list is discussed in American Diabetes Association (2010).

Chapter 11, Exercise and Weight Loss

For the importance of physical exercise in preventing or reducing the effects of disease, see Haskell et al. (2007). On the growing incidence of type 2 diabetes and the importance of diet and exercise in treating it, see Marwick et al. (2009) and Eriksson (1999). The American Diabetes Association guidelines on exercise are in Arora et al. (2009). For improved weight loss when diet and exercise are combined, see Eriksson (1999). Sarsan et al. (2006) is the source of the discussion of obesity and hypertension. Marwick et al. (2009) analyzes the role of exercise in reducing cardiovascular risk factors.

Regarding the importance of exercise to psychological health, see Sarsan et al. (2006). Haskell et al. (2007) discusses the American Heart Association recommendations on moderate- and vigorous-intensity exercise. For VO2, see Kohrt (2009). Sarsan et al. (2006) describes research on the benefits of exercise for obese women; it is the source of the statement about a study comparing strength training and aerobic exercise. The impact of aging on VO2 is discussed by Kohrt (2009). For the value of combining strength training and aerobic exercise, see Kerksick et al. (2009).

The discussion of HIIT is based largely on Teta and Teta (June 2009), with additional information from Perry (2008). See also Teta and Teta (November 2009). For stretching, see Quinn (February 16, 2010) and Witvrouw et al. (2004). The advice on how long to hold a stretch comes from the Mayo Clinic (2009).

Selections from Dr. Posner's Blog

In "Beware Hidden Sugars!" the data on sugar consumption comes from the USDA and the Sugar Association. The UN and WHO guidelines are in Casey (2003). In "Understanding Portion Control," the AICR study, USDA statistics on total daily caloric intake of Americans and American Dietetic Association advice on how to estimate portion sizes are at UPMC Nutritional Services (2010).

In "Alcohol and Weight Loss," the research on metabolic effects in men is presented by Jéquier (1999). For the Canadian study, see Tremblay et al. (1995). The study by the Royal Veterinary and Agricultural University in Denmark can be found in Raben et al. (2003).

References

American Diabetes Association (2010). Carbohydrate Counting. http://www.diabetes.org/food-and-fitness/food/planning-meals/carb-counting/.

American Heart Association (2010). *Phytochemicals and Cardiovascular Disease.* http://www.americanheart.org/presenter.jhtml?identifier=4722.

American Obesity Association (May 2, 2005). "Obesity in the U.S." http://obesity1.tempdomainname.com/subs/fastfacts/obesity_US.shtml.

American Public Health Association, Partnership for Prevention, United Health Foundation (November 2009). "The Future Cost of Obesity: National and State Estimates of the impact of Obesity on Direct Heath Care Expense." http://www.americashealthrankings.org/2009/report/Cost%20Obesity%20Report-final.pdf.

Arora, E., Shenoy, S., Sandhu, J. (2009). "Effects of Resistance Training on Metabolic Profile of Adults with Type 2 Diabetes." *Indian Journal of Medical Research* 129: 515-519.

Becker, D., Kayrooz, K., Moy, T., Yanek, L. (November 2, 2004). "Dietary Fat Patterns in Urban African-American Women." Springer Netherlands, http://www.springerlink.com/content/k6454686410584w1/.

Belluck, P. (March 17, 2005). "Children's Life Expectancy Being Cut Short by Obesity." *New York Times*, http://www.nytimes.com/2005/03/17/health/17obese.html.

Boyse, K. (May 2008). "Obesity and Overweight." University of Michigan Health Systems, http://www.med.umich.edu/yourchild/topics/obesity.htm.

Casey, J. (2003). "The Hidden Ingredient That Can Sabotage Your Diet." *WebMD*, http://www.medicinenet.com/script/main/art.asp?articlekey=56589.

Centers for Disease Control (2010). "Overweight and Obesity." http://www.cdc.gov/nccdphp/dnpa/obesity/index.htm.

Centers for Disease Control (2008). "Number of People with Diabetes Increases to 24 Million." http://www.cdc.gov/nchs/fastats/diabetes.htm.

Childhood Obesity Action Network (2007). "Expert Committee Recommendations on the Assessment, Prevention, and Treatment of Child and Adolescent Overweight and Obesity. An Implementation Guide from the Childhood Obesity Action Network." National Initiative for Children's Healthcare Quality, http://www.nichq.org/NR/rdonlyres/7CF2C1F3-4DA-4A00-AE15-4E35967F3571/5316/COANImplementationGuide-62607FINAL.pdf.

Eriksson, J.G. (1999). "Exercise and the Treatment of Type 2 Diabetes Mellitus." *Sports Medicine* 27: 381-391.

Flegal, K., Carroll, M., Ogden, C., Curtin, L. (2010). "Prevalence and Trends in Obesity among US Adults, 1999-2008." *Journal of the American Medical Association* 303(3): 235-241.

Goldstein, A. (November 17, 2009). "America's Economic Pain Brings Hunger Pangs." *Washington Post*, http://www.washingtonpost.com/wp-dyn/content/article/2009/11/16/AR2009111601598.html?wpisrc=newsletter.

Goran, M., Ball, G., Cruz, M. (2003). "Obesity and Risk of Type 2 Diabetes and Cardiovascular Disease in Children and Adolescents." *Journal of Clinical Endocrinology & Metabolism* 88(4): 1417-1427.

Haskell, W., Lee, I., Pate, R., Powell, K., Blair, S., Franklin, B., Macera, C., Heath, G., Thompson, P., Bauman, A. (2007). "Physical Activity and Public Health: Updated Recommendation for Adults from the American College of Sports Medicine and the American Heart Association." *Circulation* 116: 1081-1093.

Institute of Medicine (2004). *Dietary Reference Intakes: Water, Potassium, Sodium, Chloride, and Sulfate.* Washington, D.C.

International Food Information Council Foundation (2009). *Functional Foods Fact Sheet: Antioxidants.* http://www.foodinsight.org/Resources/Detail.aspx?topic=Functional_Foods_Fact_Sheet_Antioxidants.

Jéquier, E. (1999). JAlcohol Intake and Body Weight: A Para-dox.î *American Journal of Clinical Nutrition* 69(2): 173-174.

Kerksick, C., Thomas, A., Campbell, B., Taylor, L., Wilborn, C., Marcello, B., Roberts, M., Pfau, E., Grimstvedt, M., Opusunju, J., Magrans-Courtney, T., Rasmussen, C., Wilson, R., Kreider, R.B. (2009). "Effects of a Popular Exercise and Weight Loss Program on Weight Loss, Body Composition, Energy Expenditure and Health in Obese Women." *Nutrition & Metabolism* 6: 23-40.

Kohrt, W.M. (2009). "Menopause and Weight Gain." *Menopause Medicine* 64: 28-29.

Mahan, L.K., and Escott-Stump, S. (2008). *Krause's Food & Nutrition Therapy*, 12th ed. St. Louis.

Martlett, J., McBurney, M., Slavin, J. (2008). "Position of the American Dietetic Association: Health Implications of Dietary Fiber." *Journal of the American Dietetic Association* 108: 1716-1731.

Marwick, T., Hordern, M., Miller, T., Chyun, D., Bertoni, A., Blumenthal, R., Philippides, G, Rocchini, A. (2009). "Exercise Training for Type 2 Diabetes Mellitus: Impact on Cardiovascular Risk: A Scientific Statement from the American Heart Association." *Circulation* 119: 3244-3262.

Mayer-Davis, E., Dhawan, A., Liese, A., Teff, K., Schulz, M. (2006). "Towards Understanding of Glycemic Index and Glycemic Load in Habitual Diet: Associations with Glycemia in the Insulin Resistance Study." *British Journal of Nutrition* 95: 397.

Mayo Clinic (2009). "Stretching Like the Pros." *Mayo Clinic Health Letter* 27: 3.

McEwen, B. (2002). "Estrogen Actions throughout the Brain." *Recent Progress in Hormone Research* 57: 357-384.

Mercola, J. (January 28, 2010). "This Common Food Ingredient Can Really Mess up Your Metabolism." http://www.lewrockwell.com/orig5/mercola31.1.html.

Minority Women's Health (March 2008). "Overweight and Obesity." U.S. Department of Health and Human Services, http://www.womenshealth.gov/minority/africanamerican/obesity.cfm.

Morantz, C., and Torrey, B. (2004). "Recommendations to Reduce Obesity in Children and Adolescents." *American Family Physician* 70(12): 2377-2378.

Must, A., and Strauss, R.S. (1999). "Risks and Consequences of Childhood and Adolescent Obesity." *International Journal of Obesity* 23(2): S2-S11.

O'Callaghan, T. (2009). "Diabetes Expected to Double, Costs to Triple by 2034." http://wellness.blogs.time.com/2009/11/27/diabetes-expected-to-double-costs-to-triple-by-2034/.

Office of Minority Health (December 15, 2009). "Heart Disease and African-Americans." U.S. Department of Health and Human Services, http://minorityhealth.hhs.gov/templates/content.aspx?ID=3018.

Office of Minority Health (October 21, 2009). "African-American Profile." U.S. Department of Health and Human Services, http://minorityhealth.hhs.gov/templates/browse.aspx?lvl=2&lvlID=51.

Office of Minority Health (2009). "Obesity and African Americans." U.S. Department of Health and Human Services, http://minorityhealth.hhs.gov/templates/content.aspx?ID=6456.

Ogden, C., Carroll, M., McDowell, M., Flegal, K. (November 2007). "Obesity among Adults in the United States—No Statistically Significant Change since 2003-2004." *National Center for Health Statistics Data Brief*: 2.

Partnership to Fight Chronic Disease (2009). "The Future Costs of Obesity: National and State Estimates of the Impact of Obesity on Direct Health Care Expenses." http://www.fightchronicdisease.org/pdfs/CostofObesityReport-FINAL.pdf.

Perry, C., Heigenhauser, G., Bonen, A., Spriet, L. (2008). "High-Intensity Aerobic Interval Training Increases Fat and Carbohydrate Metabolic Capacities in Human Skeletal Muscle." *Applied Physiology, Nutrition, and Metabolism* 33(6): 1112-1123.

Posner, R. (2004). *Doctor, I Have a Chemical Imbalance: The Serotonin Story.* Burke, Virginia.

Psota, T., Gebauer, S., Kris-Etherton, P. (2006). "Dietary Omega-3 Fatty Acid Intake and Cardiovascular Risk." *American Journal of Cardiology* 98(4): 3-18.

Quinn, E. (February 16, 2010). "How to Stretch. Stretching Basics." http://www.sportsmedicine.about.com.

Raben, A., Agerholm-Larsen, L., Flint, A., Holst, J., Astrup, A. (2003). "Meals with Similar Energy Densities But Rich in Protein, Fat, Carbohydrate, or Alcohol Have Different Effects on Energy Expenditure and Substrate Metabolism But Not on Appetite and Energy Intake." *American Journal of Clinical Nutrition* 77(1): 91-100.

Rao, G. (July 1, 2009). "Childhood Obesity: Highlights of AMA Expert Committee Recommendations." *American Family Physician*: 34, 37.

Sarsan, A., Ardic, F., Ozgen, M., Topuz, O. (2006). "The Effects of Aerobic and Resistance Exercises in Obese Women." *Clinical Rehabilitation* 20: 773-782.

Simopoulos, P. (2008). "The Importance of the Omega-6/Omega-3 Fatty Acid Ratio in Cardiovascular Disease and Other Chronic Diseases." *Experimental Biology and Medicine* 233: 674-688.

Teta, J., and Teta, K. (November 2009). "Revisiting Exercise for Weight Loss." *Townsend Letter:* 114-115.

Teta, J., and Teta, K. (June 2009). "Interval Exercise as Treatment for Cardiovascular Diseases?" *Townsend Letter*: 100-101.

Tremblay, A., Wouters, E., Wenker, M., St-Pierre, S., Bouchard, C., Després, J.P. (1995). "Alcohol and a High-Fat Diet: A Combination Favoring Overfeeding." *American Journal of Clinical Nutrition* 62: 639–644.

UPMC Nutritional Services (2010). "Understanding Portion Control."
http://nutritionservices.upmc.com/NutritionArticles/Habits/Portions.htm.

Westman, E., Feinman, R., Mavropoulos, J., Vernon, M., Volek, J., Wortman, J., Yancy, W., Phinney, S. (2007). "Low-Carbohydrate Nutrition and Metabolism." *American Journal of Clinical Nutrition* 86(2): 276-284.
http://www.ajcn.org/cgi/content/full/86/2/276.

Wilson, G. (2008). *Carbohydrates, Proteins, and Fats.*
http://www.merck.com/mmhe/sec12/ch152/ch152b.html.

Witvrouw, E., Mahieu, N., Danneels, L., McNair, P. (2004). "Stretching and Injury Prevention: An Obscure Relationship." *Sports Medicine* 34: 443-449.

About the Authors

Robert B. Posner, M.D., is the Founder and Medical Director of the Serotonin-Plus Weight Loss Program. Dr. Posner graduated with Phi Beta Kappa honors from Binghamton State University in 1977 and then attended Downstate Medical School in New York City, graduating in 1981. In 1984, he became certified as a Diplomate of the American Board of Internal Medicine. During his active duty tour in the U.S. Navy, he was selected to interview for the position of physician to President Reagan as well as physician to Congress. Dr. Posner was voted Teacher of the Year by the Jacksonville Naval Hospital family practice residents in 1986 and was awarded the Navy Achievement Medal in 1988. He has been in private practice in the northern Virginia area for 21 years, and has taught internal medicine residents from Georgetown University and medical students from such institutions as the Medical College of Virginia.

Dr. Posner researched and patented the **Serotonin Formula™,** a unique oral serotonin supplement for weight loss (U.S. Patent Number 6,017,946). He has also investigated serotonin replacement for serotonin imbalance conditions such as depression, chronic fatigue, migraine headaches, premenstrual syndrome, fibromyalgia and myofascial pain syndrome. His book, *Doctor, I Have a Chemical Imbalance: The Serotonin Story,* was published in 2004. Dr. Posner is expanding the Serotonin-Plus Weight Loss Program nationally and the SP Program is currently in 23 states and growing.

Dr. Posner is an avid sports enthusiast and can be found on the tennis courts or running in his free time.

Donna L. Eckenrode, MPAS, PA-C, is Serotonin-Plus USA Director of Clinical Training. After graduating from Saint Francis University in 2003 with a master's in physician assistant sciences, she worked as a physician assistant at a family practice in Reston, Virginia, before changing her focus to neurology. As part of one of the largest neurology practices in northern Virginia, she cared for patients with multiple neurological conditions including Parkinson's disease, multiple sclerosis, seizures and neuropathy. Following the birth of her daughter, she took a position with Dr. Robert Posner at Serotonin-Plus Weight Loss, where she has enjoyed working for the past year. Working at Serotonin-Plus Weight Loss has afforded her the opportunity to integrate her lifelong interest in fitness and nutrition with her professional role as a physician assistant.

Julia Yuskavage, M.S., R.D., is the Registered Dietitian and Director of Nutritional Programs at Serotonin-Plus USA. She received her degree in dietetics from James Madison University in 2006, completed her master's of science in nutrition at Virginia Tech in 2008, and graduated from the Virginia Tech Dietetic Internship program in 2009.

Julia Yuskavage has played an intricate role in fine-tuning the nutritional program at Serotonin-Plus by staying abreast of the latest nutritional science and using it to safely maximize our patients' weight loss. She has a flair for cooking and can often be found testing healthy and flavorful new recipes for her patients and co-workers, investigating new food products at health food stores or pursuing her daily fitness routine of jumping rope and strength training.

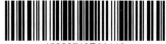

Made in the USA
Middletown, DE
16 July 2017